A Century
of Caring

A History of
Anne Arundel
Medical Center
1902 - 2002

Catherine H. Avery
Jane W. McWilliams

AMERICANS HAVE MANY QUALITIES THAT SET THEM APART FROM THE
CITIZENS OF THE REST OF THE WORLD, BUT NONE IS MORE TYPICAL
AND DISTINCTIVE THAN THEIR GENUINE AND INTENSE CONCERN WITH
MATTERS OF HEALTH.

REAR ADMIRAL F. C. GREAVES, USN
At the ground-breaking for the Summerfield Baldwin, Jr.
Memorial Wing Anne Arundel General Hospital
November 6, 1952

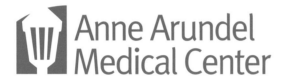

Anne Arundel
Medical Center

2001 Medical Parkway
Annapolis, Maryland 21401
www.aahs.org

Assistance in the research and preparation
for this book was provided by Anne Arundel
Medical Center Public Relations and the
Center for the Study of Local Issues, Anne
Arundel Community College.

Hardcover ISBN 0-9633013-1-4
Softcover ISBN 0-9633013-2-2

CONTENTS

To the Tretten Family,

I hope you enjoy this history of AAMC. Your Dad was very much a part of it! I had the privilege of coming here as a young administrator in 1972. One of my first impressions was how competent, compassionate and caring a Medical Staff. Your Dad was one of the main reasons for those impressions. No one was more skilled in his specialty or more caring about his patients than your Dad.

I had the opportunity to reconnect as the years have gone by, and he came back for his own health care. On his last few visits I had the opportunity to visit and a chance to thank him, to tell him what he had meant to me personally. Any praise he always wanted to reflect on others. That of course was Gene's modesty.

Your Dad was very special! I will always remember a gentle man to whom this community owes so much. My best to you and thanks for letting me share a few memories.

Chip

6

Commemorating Our Centennial

How does one measure the value of an institution? By the number of people it affects? By its sheer longevity? Its ability to meet community needs? Or a long-standing reputation for trust, integrity and commitment?

By any measure, the commemoration of the founding of Anne Arundel Medical Center gives us reason to pause. It's a time for reflection. That indomitable force that swept through Annapolis at the turn of the century was created by a core of strong-willed women who determined that this town could no longer be without a hospital. It was their pioneer spirit that helped found the Annapolis Emergency Hospital on February 17, 1902. And, in a pattern of giving that would mark this institution forever, a handful of leading citizens donated their time and financial support to open the doors to the hospital's first patient on July 18, 1902.

This also is a time to celebrate. The first 100 years record sentinel achievements in healthcare for this community and for the nation. Hundreds of thousands of lives began here. Thousands of people have made their livelihoods here, supporting their families and their own communities. The hospital's impact on this region has been profound and long lasting.

And, perhaps most importantly, it's a time to give thanks. The story of Anne Arundel Medical Center over 10 decades is the story of many, many people who have devoted their lives to its success. From its early founding by the "Lady Board of Managers" to the men and women who serve on today's Board of Trustees, Foundation Board and other volunteer boards and committees, to the 600 members of our medical staff, 2,000 employees, 900 members of our Auxiliary, and the

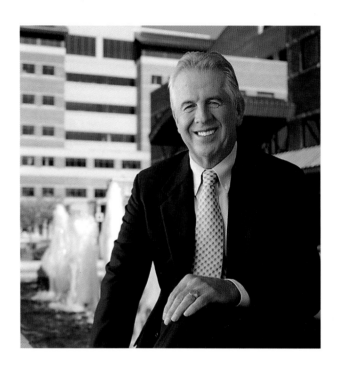

scores of leading contributors and thousands more who give whatever they can, this hospital is a tribute to the best in people.

Finally, this is a time to look forward. A century of achievement sets a challenge to perform even better in the next. Given the solid foundation this organization enjoys—and the will of so many dedicated people—Anne Arundel Medical Center offers a bright and promising future for the patients and families who seek its care. The new Acute Care Pavilion that rises on the Medical Park campus opens our new century as a symbol of what philanthropy, trust and commitment can achieve not only for today, but also for our future.

Martin L. Doordan
President
Anne Arundel Health System

Foreword

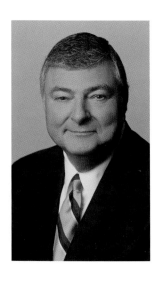

What follows in these remarkable pages is more than the story of the founding and growth of a hospital. It also is the chronicle of a community's pride, vision, courage, compassion and generosity.

Anne Arundel Medical Center, by its very existence, makes many promises—most of them unspoken—to its community. But the women and men who lead, staff and volunteer at this very special place keep those promises again and again every day. For a century, they have created a chain of memories in the lives of millions of people for whom they have made a profound difference. Here are just a few of those promises:

That the doors will never close...that whatever the challenges, crises, the community's new and changing needs, the hospital will find a way to meet the challenges and fulfill those needs.

That for everyone who comes to the hospital's doors in need—no matter who they are or what has happened to them—the people of Anne Arundel Medical Center will do their best for them.

That everyone who is a part of this special place does their work as a calling to the service of others with the highest ethic and spirit of compassion. That the hospital's mission is not only to treat the ill and injured and offer care and hope to them and their families, but also to make the community a healthier, safer place.

Those promises and all of the others are part of the legacy that has its roots on Franklin Street in downtown Annapolis. With the hospital's move to Medical Park, those promises have been preserved and built upon by the thousands of dedicated people who have given part of their lives to the medical center.

Today, Anne Arundel Medical Center is a respected regional medical center, bringing the most advanced medical care available to a vast new community. It is investing in the newest technologies, attracting some of the most skilled caregivers from across America and even around the world, and bringing vital facilities and services close to home.

But as much as Anne Arundel Medical Center has changed from its birth 100 years ago, some things remain the same. You can see it in the faces on the pages in this book and you can see it in the faces of the staff that makes it the very special place it is today. This book tells the real story of this hospital, its soul and its mission—promises made, promises kept.

Dick Davidson

Richard J. Davidson
President
American Hospital Association

The new Acute Care Pavilion stands like a beacon of light, welcoming residents from throughout the region to enter its doors and receive state-of-the-art care in a healing environment. The building has six patient care floors and 182 private patient rooms, and is designed to improve care in every way.

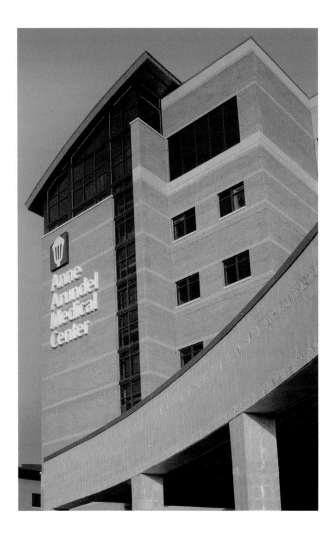

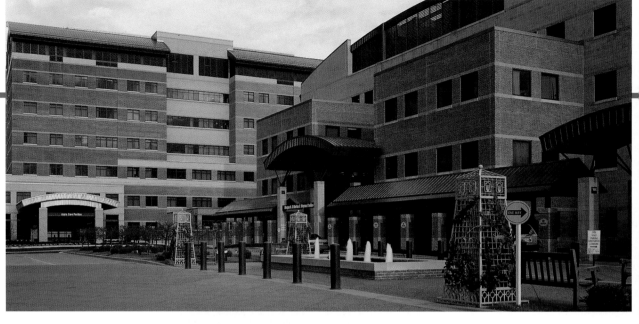

A view of the campus looking toward the new Acute Care Pavilion.

The Clatanoff Pavilion lobby (right) offers an elegant entry to the patient care rooms upstairs, which quickly convert from hotel-like luxury to high-tech efficiency (below) for maternity patients.

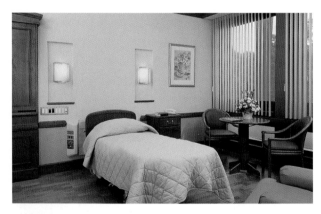

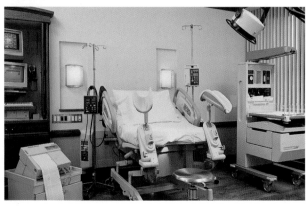

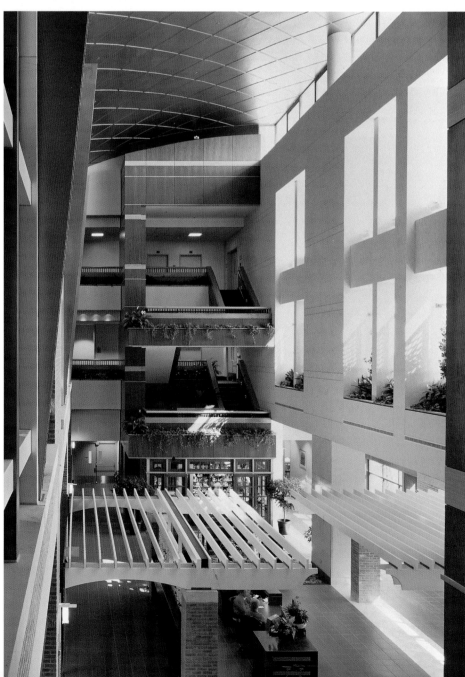

10

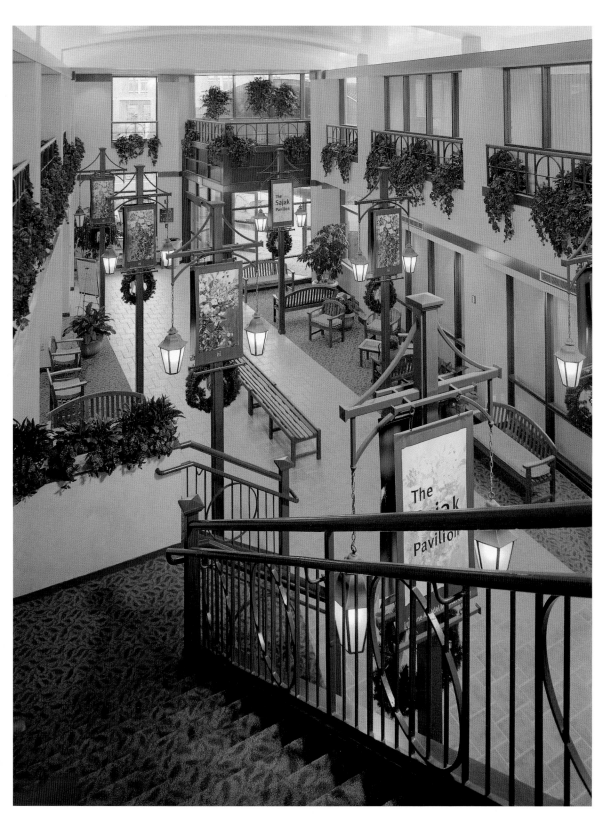

The Sajak Pavilion, opened in March 2001, features an attractive, light-filled lobby adjacent to the Breast Center (below). The six-floor building also houses ambulatory services, doctors' offices and hospital administration.

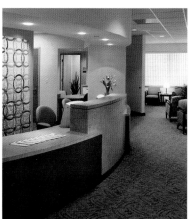

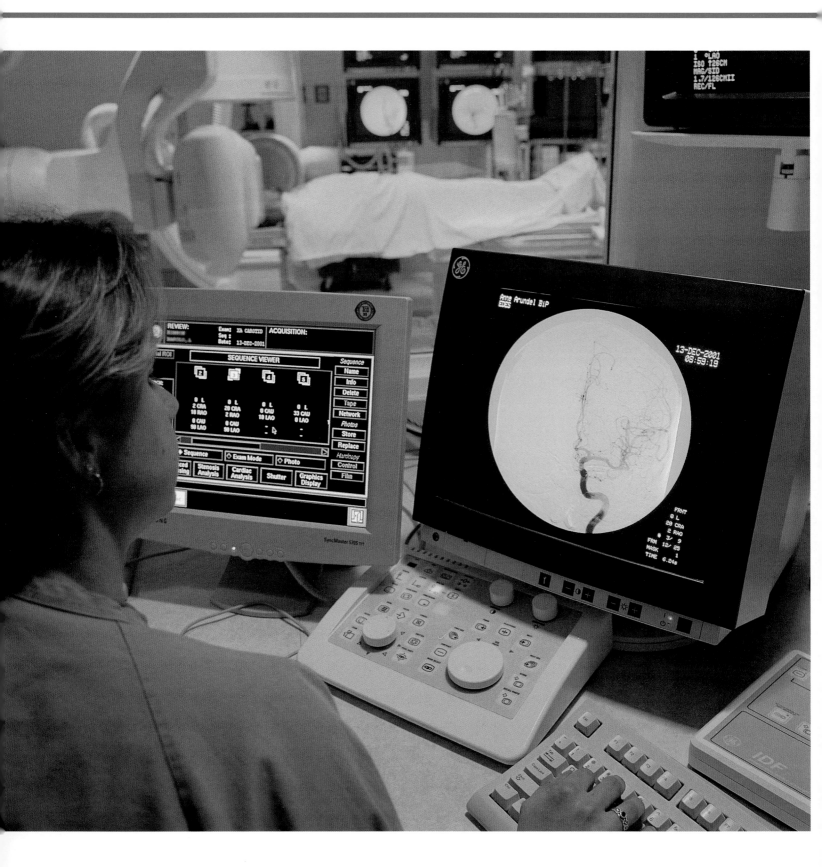

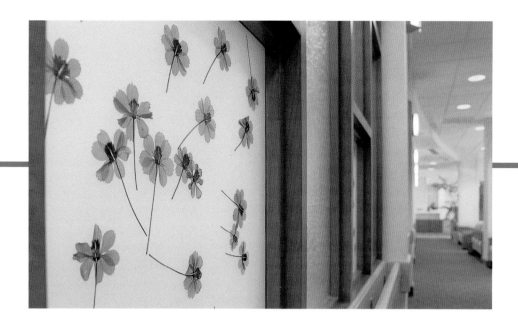

The hospital incorporates all the latest technologies, including sophisticated vascular imaging (left). The emergency department (right) is fully equipped for up-to-the-minute testing and monitoring in a comforting environment.

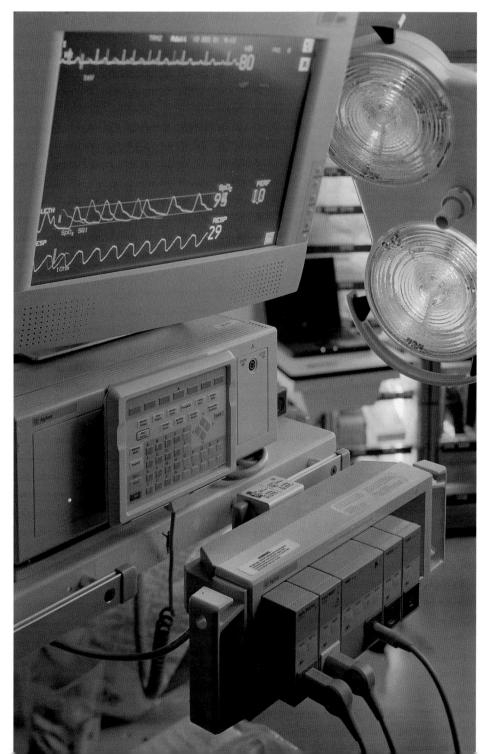

The Meditation Center offers an oasis with a stained glass window by local artist Bobbie Burnett, donated by the Auxiliary. The Garden Café (below) provides a place to catch a quick bite in a pleasing environment.

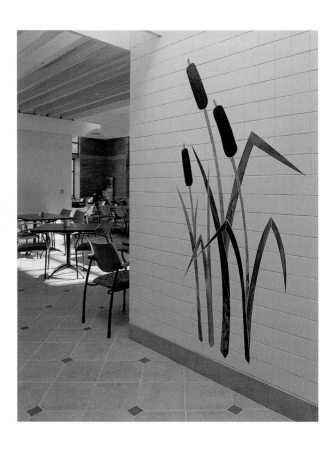

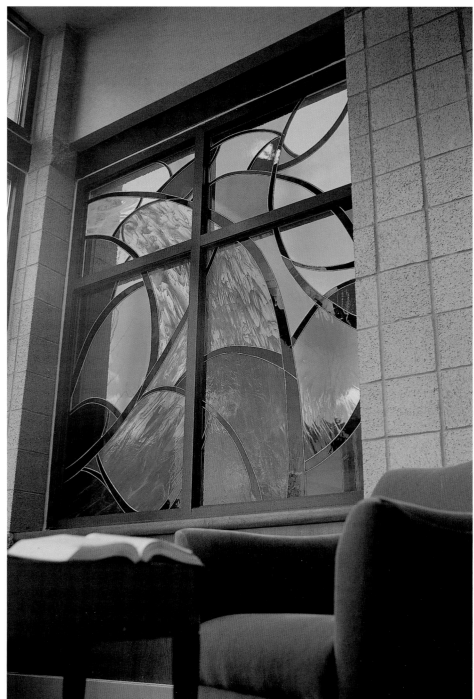

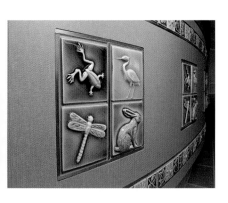

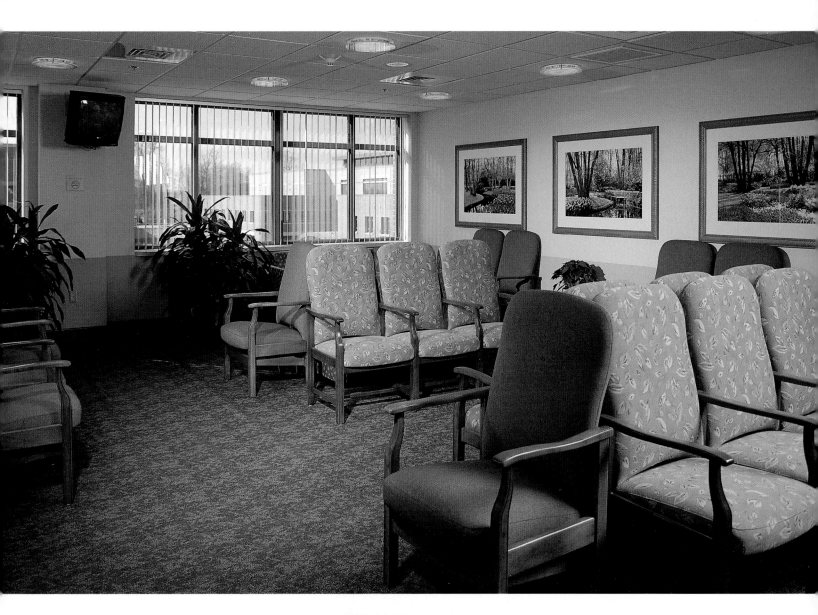

Family comfort is a priority at the new Acute Care Pavilion. Spacious, well-furnished waiting areas are strategically located. Special touches—colorful wall tiles and lively floor decorations (top and right)—contribute to the healing environment throughout the hospital. A nature theme prevails, supported by soft lights, natural colors and carpeted hallways.

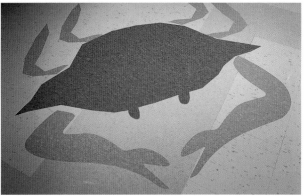

My grandparents moved to Annapolis in 1901 and opened a bakery on Main Street.

They had a bakery in Westminster before, but they came here because they thought it would be a good place to set up business. Annapolis was much more up-and-coming than Westminster.

Annapolis was a very small town then and Sunday dinner was the big event of the week. Everyone got dressed up for the Sunday meal; the whole family got together and guests were invited. As a single woman working in Annapolis, this was a coveted invitation for my mother. The other big activity was to go to the beach—they would go to Bay Ridge or to the South River near Route 2—and wear these very elaborate bathing costumes.

My mother and my aunt both were nurses at the hospital. In fact, my aunt introduced my mother to my father. My mother lived in the Nurses' Home until she got married, and then she had to quit; the hospital wouldn't accept married nurses then.

All the nurses worked 12-hour shifts. They were paid $100 a month, but that included meals and lodging so it was a pretty good deal. The nurses did a little bit of everything—wash patients, empty bedpans, change beds, give medications, assist with deliveries, work in the operating room. There were no nurses' aides. My mother said that sometimes she had to deliver babies when the doctor couldn't make it to the hospital on time!

The nurses thought the doctors were next to God. They were much loved— I remember Dr. Purvis spoken of with great respect. The patients were very appreciative of the care they received. But some things were different back then—I remember hearing that the nurses would wash patients' upper bodies, and then give patients the washcloth and instruct them, 'Now you go as far down as possible.'

I was born at the hospital in 1928— actually I was born in the Nurses' Home, because of the hospital fire. I've had several surgeries there, too. It's been a real part of my life.

Perspective...

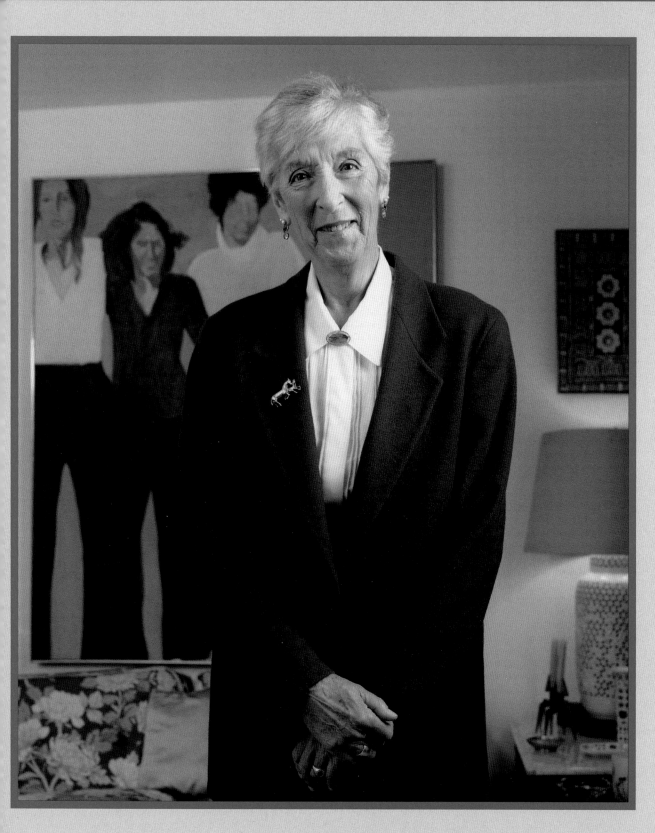

Peg Wohlgemuth Burroughs

Born in Nurses' Home, 1928

Grandaughter of Annapolis business owners

Daughter of Veronica Fitzgerald, R.N., hospital nurse, c.1918-1923

Niece of Margaret Wohlgemuth, R.N., hospital superintendent 1915-17, 1919-23

As the 19th century drew to a close, Americans faced the 20th with a sense of optimism and anticipation. It was an exciting time, a time when nearly everything seemed possible, when the miracles of science promised to contribute to the public good as well as to private profit. Recent discoveries and inventions enabled people for the first time to control their environment and perhaps even their destiny. There was electricity to light the darkness with the flip of a switch, the telephone to summon help or friends, indoor plumbing, central heat, the automobile to open new avenues to adventure and success.

In medicine, the development of the germ theory in the last quarter of the 19th century led to dramatic progress in identifying the causes of disease and easing suffering through clinical diagnosis and sterile surgery. New inventions such as the thermometer and the X-ray offered physicians methods of quantifying and standardizing diagnoses. By 1900, the killer diseases of the day were on notice. The organisms that produced tuberculosis and cholera had been identified. There were serological tests for typhoid and an antitoxin for diphtheria. The ancient belief that sickness came to those whose way of life or general physical state encouraged it was challenged by the awareness that germ-produced disease could threaten anyone who drank contaminated water, for instance, or came in contact with an infected person.

Recognition of the role of microorganisms in illness increased public concern with sanitation. Florence Nightingale's lessons on cleanliness and ventilation in the sickroom began to be applied to living conditions in general. The prospect that diseases such as cholera and typhoid could be prevented, or at least controlled, by attention to the physical envi-

ronment brought new hope and energy to a growing public health movement uniting scientists, doctors, politicians, public administrators and laymen (and women).

With the new century upon them, the people of America looked ahead to the serious work of making their communities better places in which to live. They believed theirs to be the best country in the world and they were filled with pride.

The United States had emerged from the Spanish-American War in 1898 as a nation to be reckoned with on the international scene and with territories in the Caribbean and Pacific that required a mighty navy to secure. For Annapolis, home to the U.S. Naval Academy, this new emphasis on a large naval force promised a bustle and excitement that would fulfill the longings of restive city fathers.

Annapolis had always been a government town. Ever since the capital of Maryland moved to Annapolis in 1695, the town's focus had been politics. The state government, together with the county and city governments, employed enough of the populace to cushion economic hard times. And, since 1845, the Naval Academy's presence had given the small town on the Severn a place in the national consciousness. Annapolitans were proud of the academy and their association with the officers of the U.S. Navy.

Yet, since its pre-Revolutionary glory days, Annapolis had been eclipsed by Baltimore, its large and powerful urban neighbor to the north. By the late 19th century, Annapolitans feared themselves completely out of the mainstream of industrial America. The city had rail and boat connections to Washington and Baltimore, a small glassworks in nearby

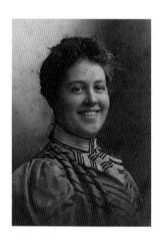

Emma N. Feldmeyer, one of the founding members of the Annapolis Emergency Hospital Association and treasurer from 1905 to 1919.

THE COTTAGE HOSPITAL
The Beginning to 1910

Eastport and the biennial meetings of the legislature; but outside of government, its major industry was seafood-oriented: the collection, processing and shipping of the Chesapeake Bay's harvest. Now, with the dawn of the new century, Annapolis embraced the prospect of importance by installing a new sewer system and paving West Street from Church Circle to Colonial Avenue. Simultaneously, major building projects were begun by both the state of Maryland and the federal government.

In 1900, the state legislature authorized construction of a building on Bladen Street, between State Circle and College Avenue, to house the Court of Appeals. Work began in 1901 and was followed by authorizations in 1902 for a new state heating plant and an annex to the State House. Construction on these began immediately.

The new Post Office Building on Church Circle, built in 11 months in 1901, was a source of pride for Annapolis residents, but the federal projects at the Naval Academy captured their full attention. The hodgepodge of 19th-century buildings was to be demolished and replaced with massive and beautiful stone and brick structures, designed by architect Ernest Flagg and appropriate to the

The property of florist Edwin A. Seidewitz, facing a path that would become Cathedral Street, before 1891.

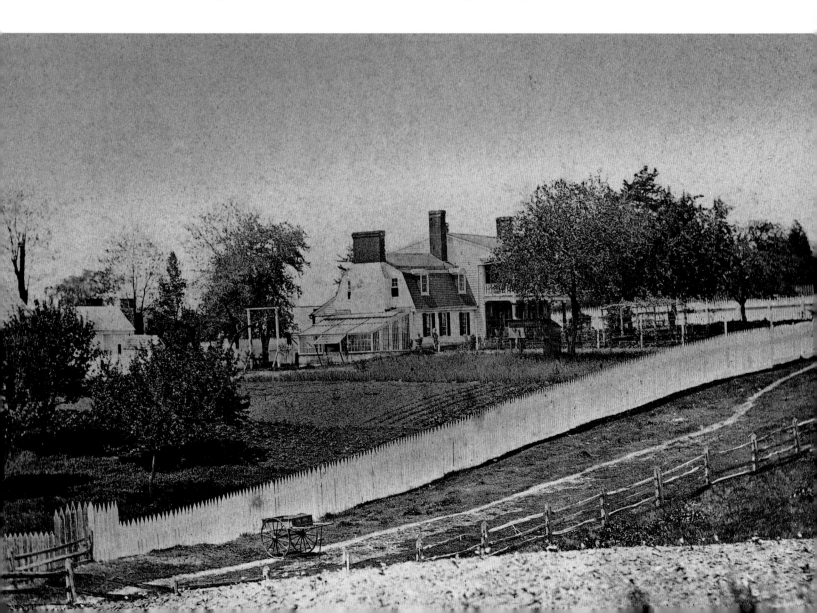

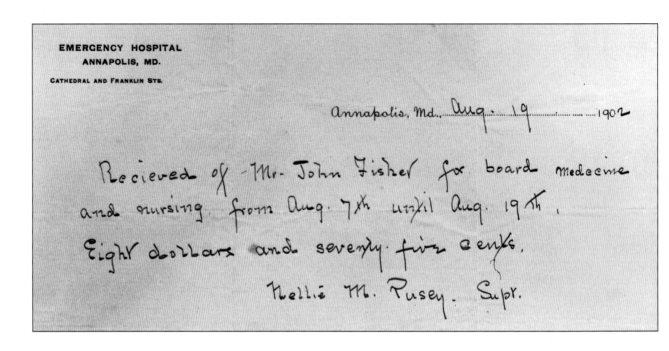

A receipt for a hospital bill, 1902.

EMERGENCY HOSPITAL
ANNAPOLIS, MD.

CATHEDRAL AND FRANKLIN STS.

Annapolis, Md., Aug. 19 1902

Recieved of Mr. John Fisher for board medecine and nursing from Aug. 7th until Aug. 19th. Eight dollars and seventy-five cents.

Nellie M. Rusey. Supt.

education of naval officers in a nation that was asserting itself as a sea power. Work began first on a great armory, Dahlgren Hall, and in 1902 the foundation was laid for Bancroft Hall, to be the largest dormitory in the world. Also scheduled were new classroom buildings, a power house, officers' housing, a boathouse, naval hospital and an impressive new chapel to be topped with a golden dome.

Seemingly overnight, Annapolis was overflowing with stone masons and construction workers, some of whom brought their families with them. With the increased demand for housing and commodities, private enterprise flourished. A hotel was built next to the Annapolis and Baltimore Short Line Railroad station on Bladen Street and another, called Carvel Hall, was created from the old Paca House on Prince George Street.

By the end of 1901, the Annapolis *Maryland Republican* could say:

"Probably no city in the country, certainly no city of the size of Annapolis, has changed so much in the past two years. One who has not seen the city for this length of time would surely be amazed at its changed condition. The splendid buildings in course of erection at the Naval Academy, the fine State building now going up, the handsome post office, just completed, the smooth vitrified brick streets and the perfect sewers have made a new Annapolis. The change in the material condition of Annapolis is also working a change in the thoughts and habits of its people and there is no question that its people are beginning to realize that the twentieth century is opening a new future for their city, a future undreamed of a few years ago."

The local papers, the *Maryland Republican* and the *Evening Capital*, followed the building boom with almost daily reports of progress and front-page stories of the accidents that inevitably accompanied it. When a scaffold gave way at the new Naval Academy boathouse and Patrick Burns fell 40 feet to his death in December 1901, the *Evening Capital* reported the event in gruesome detail. When Charles Fisher was struck in the eye with a piece of iron pipe at the new power plant, the *Evening Capital* elaborated on his treatment at the Presbyterian Eye, Ear and Throat Hospital in Baltimore and noted that he had a wife and five children. Injuries occurred almost daily and the newspapers' stories usually cited the place of treatment: a Baltimore hospital, a local hotel, the Naval Academy hospital, at home. Watermen with no family in town were often taken to the city jail for treatment.

Health—or rather, sickness—appeared to be much on the minds of the editors. They faithfully recorded the statistics of city health officer Dr. John Ridout for 1901: 171 births, 170 deaths (January 13, 1902); the operations performed on local residents: "Mr. Onofrio Geraci is quite sick at St. Joseph's Hospital, Baltimore, where he recently had an operation performed for cancer of the jaw" (January 14, 1902); and the condition of convalescents: "Delegate T.J.J. Smoot, a member of the House from Charles County, who has been so very ill and confined to his room at the Chesapeake House on Main Street, is very much improved and able to sit up" (January 21, 1902). These items of local interest shared the *Capital's* pages with graphic advertisements for patent medicines: Dr. Pierce's Favorite Prescription for "womanly weakness"; Hood's Sarsaparilla for "scrofula, glandular tumors, abscesses, pimples, sore ears, rickets"; Botanic Blood Balm for blood poi-

soning and cancer; Fletcher's Castoria; and Scott's Emulsion, which, exclaimed its promoters, "feeds the body, starves the microbes!. . .We can't expect to understand all about these germs and microbes the doctors talk of. They say that one kind causes consumption. Consumption microbes feed on weak lungs. Perhaps that is so. At any rate we know that Scott's Emulsion has a peculiar action on the lungs which gives the lungs new life and vigor," (November 27, 1901).

On January 25, 1902, the *Evening Capital* reported that the ladies of Annapolis were interested in establishing a local hospital. Because of the "numerous accidents" during the construction of the Naval Academy, the wife of the superintendent was among those promoting the cause.

As the reporter acknowledged, the idea of a community hospital for Annapolis was not new. In the mid-1870s, Agnes Randall and Eliza Lockwood Sigsbee had raised $1,000 from benefit entertainments toward a hospital fund. Both women, then in their twenties, were Annapolis natives: Agnes was the daughter of lawyer Alexander Randall, U. S. congressman and attorney general of Maryland and president of Farmers National Bank; and Eliza was the daughter of Henry H. Lockwood, a professor at the Naval Academy and a brigadier general during the Civil War. Agnes Randall married, in 1879, Dr. Thomas B. Brune, a Baltimore surgeon. Eliza Sigsbee's husband was commanding officer of the *Maine* when it exploded in Havana Harbor, February 15, 1898, thus setting off the Spanish-American War.

There is some evidence that a "cottage hospital" did operate for a brief period in the late 1870s, but by 1887 the remaining money in

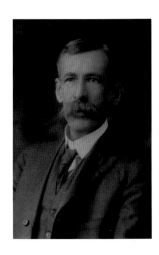

Dr. William S. Welch, a graduate of the University of Maryland Medical School, was the father and grandfather of physicians on the hospital's staff.

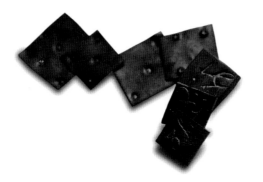

the Cottage Hospital Fund was given to the Hospital Club of St. Anne's Church.

The Hospital Club had been formed in April 1887 by the women of St. Anne's Church in response to an article by Harriet McEwen Kimball in the *Churchman*, an Episcopal publication. Mrs. Kimball advocated the distribution of furniture and clothing useful to the sick and assistance to the sick in obtaining proper nourishment and medicine. The women of St. Anne's corresponded with Mrs. Kimball and, encouraged by their rector, Rev. William S. Southgate, began these good works in Annapolis. Collecting dues of 10 cents a month from club members, they purchased and gathered suitable equipment and organized home visits to the sick.

Among those involved were Agnes Randall Brune's stepmother, Elizabeth Blanchard Randall, her sister Katherine W. Randall and her half-sister Elizabeth Blanchard Randall. The club's treasurer was Miss Nannie S. Stockett, the organist at St. Anne's. The furniture and supplies for distribution, lodged in a storeroom in the Randall home off College Avenue, included mattresses, bed linens, clothing for the sick, "invalids' chairs," hot water bags and old linens.

The club kept careful records and printed its annual reports in pamphlet form. Members made more than 300 visits to about 60 needy sick people a year between 1887 and 1895. Contributions from the St. Anne's Alms Fund and memberships and donations averaged about $100 a year during this period.

When an Annapolis hospital was again discussed in the winter of 1901–1902, there was talk of organizing it under the wing of the Hospital Club or the Associated Charities of Annapolis. The need for a facility to treat the injured was clear, as was the need for the facility to be supported, at least in part, by the state and local governments. The county delegation to the General Assembly was sympathetic to the cause and they were joined by Naval Academy personnel and the construction contractors of both state and federal buildings.

On February 8, 1902, about 35 interested citizens gathered at an organizational meeting chaired by Mayor Charles A. DuBois and appointed a Board of Managers to form a corporation. Nine days later, on February 17, 1902, incorporation papers were filed in Anne Arundel County Circuit Court for the Annapolis Emergency Hospital Association with the stated purpose of "establishing and conducting an Emergency Hospital in the City of Annapolis." Named in the document as a Board of Managers for the first year were Charles A. DuBois, Evelyn Wainwright, Anna L. Cresap, Katherine Walton, Phoebe E. Martin, Emma N. Feldmeyer, Catharine C. McComas, Katherine D. Andrews, Emma Abbott Gage, Lillian W. Clark and Katherine S. Culver. The first officers of the corporation were Mayor DuBois, president; Mrs. Cresap, vice president; Miss Andrews, treasurer; and Mrs. Gage, secretary.

These "ladies of the board" represented local churches, businesses and the academy. Most were native Annapolitans in their late thirties or early forties, the wives or daughters of local businessmen and professionals. Anna Cresap, a Catholic, was the recent widow of retired Navy Lt. Comdr. James C. Cresap; Katherine Walton, an artist of considerable repute, was the daughter of local physician Dr. Henry Roland Walton; Phoebe E. Martin's husband was seafood wholesaler John W. Martin; Emma N. Feldmeyer, a Methodist, was the wife of dentist George T. Feldmeyer; Catherine C. McComas was the daughter of Navy Paymaster James D. Murray and wife of Rev. Joseph P. McComas, rector of St. Anne's; Kate Andrews, a Methodist, was one of the five spinster Andrews sisters of Maryland Avenue whose father, James Andrews, was a local merchant; Emma Abbott Gage, daughter of William M. Abbott, owner and publisher of the *Evening Capital*, was herself the paper's local editor; and Katherine Culver, at 54 probably the oldest of the group, was the wife of George A. Culver, cashier of Farmers National Bank. Evelyn Wainwright and Lillian W. Clark were the wives of the Naval Academy superintendent and chaplain, respectively.

The board turned immediately to representatives of the state, county and city governments for aid. On February 25, 1902, Anne Arundel County Delegate James R. Brashears introduced a bill in the House for annual appropriations to the new hospital. The county commissioners and city aldermen followed suit. By early spring, the Annapolis Emergency Hospital Association had secured pledges of $1,500 annually for two years from the state, $500 from the county and $150 from the city of Annapolis.

Civic and fraternal organizations, churches and individuals responded quickly to the board's request for donations and pledges. Among the first contributors were the Universal Lodge No. 14 AF and AM ("the colored lodge of Masons"); P. J. Carlin Co., contractors for the armory and boathouse at the academy; the Annapolis Baptist Church; and the academy's Circle Club, which donated the proceeds of its production of "HMS Pinafore" at the Opera House—$280— to the hospital fund.

By mid-March, with fundraising well under-

way and the government appropriations assured, the question of a location for the hospital solved itself with the offer of former mayor Edwin A. Seidewitz to sell the association a part of his property on Franklin and Cathedral streets for what the *Evening Capital* called the "very moderate price of $3,500." Edwin A. Seidewitz was a florist with an extensive nursery operation in the block between Franklin and Cathedral streets and a cove of Spa Creek. He supplied flowers for Annapolis weddings and events and was successful enough to open florist shops in Arlington, Virginia and Baltimore, where he was living in 1902.

At the time Seidewitz's property was being considered by the new hospital board, there were two dwellings on the Franklin Street side of the land and greenhouses along Cathedral Street and across the interior of the lot. Acton Cove, an arm of Spa Creek, intruded into the property at its southeasternmost corner and neither South nor Shaw streets was cut through to their present intersection. The original line of Doctor (now Franklin) Street south of Cathedral lay about 30 feet to the east of its present path, but by the mid-1890s it had been relocated, widened and renamed.

It was the larger of the two houses that the hospital board considered suitable. This white frame building had a two-story main block facing Cathedral Street with porches across the front and a one-and-a-half story gambrel-roofed wing to the east. In the 18th century, the property had been the residence of Dr. Richard Tootell, a physician during the Revolutionary era. A description of his house in 1798 matches that of the gambrel-roofed wing of the Seidewitz house and it is tempting to assume that this old dwelling had seen the patients of an earlier time.

With the state's promise of the necessary $3,500, Annapolis Emergency Hospital Association purchased about a half acre—20,400 square feet—at the corner of Franklin and Cathedral streets, including the dwelling, from Seidewitz on May 31, 1902. Title to the land was vested in the state of Maryland, but the transfer was "for the purposes of an Emergency Hospital at Annapolis."

The board was delighted. The site, the managers said, was "peculiarly well adapted to their needs, being sunny and elevated and commanding a fine view of Spa Creek and so situated as to receive the unobstructed breezes from the Bay—thus making it an ideal spot for a Hospital and capable of future growth." Community associations, individuals and the class of 1902 of the Naval Academy offered to equip rooms.

The physicians of Annapolis met in early May at the Seidewitz house to organize the medical staff and suggest improvements that would turn the former residence into a working hospital. Meeting with them were Mayor DuBois of the Board of Managers and three Baltimore doctors who were elected consulting physicians.

The local doctors who would constitute the first staff included Drs. William Bishop, Washington Clement Claude, Frank H. Thompson, Henry Roland Walton and William S. Welch of Annapolis; Dr. William G. Ridout and his son Dr. John Ridout, public health officer for the city; Dr. George Wells and young Dr. Sewell S. Hepburn of south county; and Dr. T. C. Walton of the Naval Academy. The consulting doctors from Baltimore were Dr. Frank Robert Smith, associate professor of medicine at Johns Hopkins Medical School

and part-time staff member at Johns Hopkins Hospital; Dr. Thomas S. Cullen, associate professor of gynecology at Hopkins Medical School and later head of the department of gynecology at Johns Hopkins Hospital; and Dr. Joseph C. Bloodgood, associate professor of surgery at Hopkins Medical School and later head of surgical pathology at Johns Hopkins Hospital.

The arrangement whereby big-city physicians served as consultants to local family practitioners was common in community hospitals at this time and for many years to come.

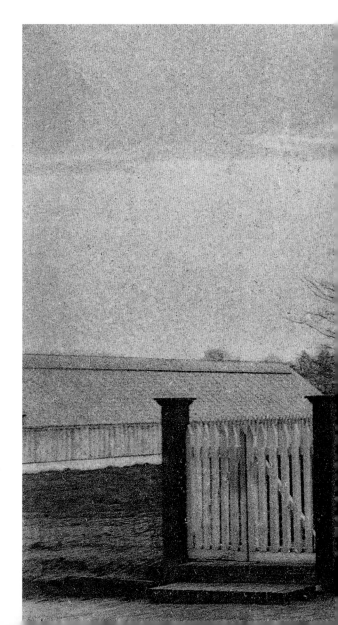

Annapolis was fortunate to be located within easy traveling distance of large teaching hospitals and drew principally from the staffs of the University of Maryland and Johns Hopkins in Baltimore, the latter of which had opened its medical school in 1893. The local doctors, many of them trained at the University of Maryland Medical School, were primarily family physicians who cared for their patients on a day-to-day basis. They traveled the city and county in horse and buggy, making their rounds of home visits and treating the sick who came to their home offices. They routinely performed house-call surgery on kitchen tables under conditions that would be viewed with horror by the operating room staffs of today.

Medical care in 1902 had not progressed much beyond the mid-19th-century strictures of Florence Nightingale: proper nourishment, good nursing care and bed rest. Surgical procedures had, however, made great strides since Joseph Lister's work with atmospheric disinfection in the 1870s. Antiseptic surgery, as practiced daily by the doctors of municipal hospitals, promised recovery rates unheard of a quarter century before.

The Seidewitz house in its new role as the Annapolis Emergency Hospital, c.1905.

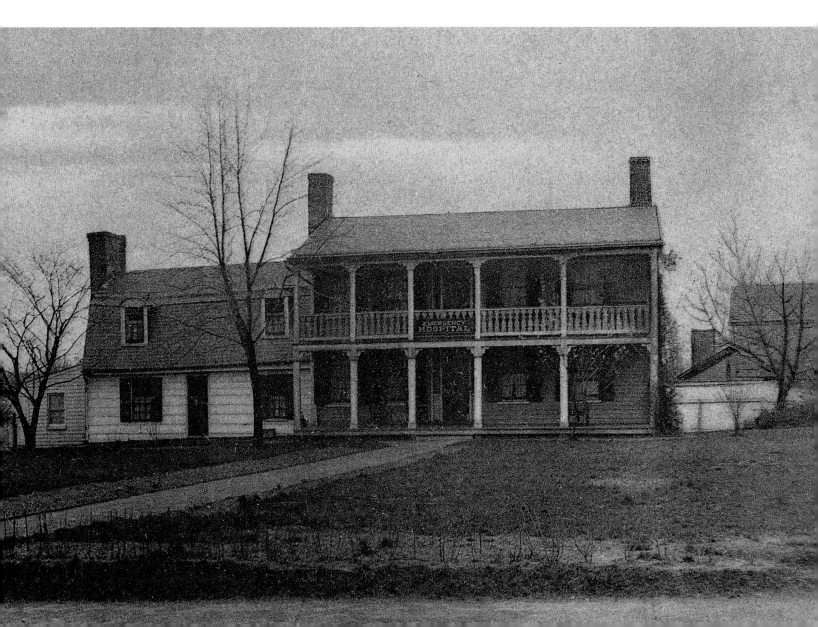

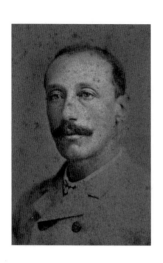

Dr. William Bishop, a graduate of Howard University School of Medicine, was a prominent physician and Annapolis resident of African-American descent.

The Annapolis Emergency Hospital's consultants, with their exposure to the wide range of illnesses in an urban area and their close association with the latest advances in medical science at teaching hospitals, brought both experience and knowledge to Annapolis. The patients of the Annapolis Emergency Hospital would have the best of both worlds: the most up-to-date procedures as practiced by a well-trained surgeon and their own familiar family doctor close at hand, often administering the anesthesia.

It is no wonder the Annapolis physicians were happy to participate in the preparations for a new hospital in their town. Not only would it provide a sanitary, well-ordered nursing environment for their patients and a properly equipped operating room for surgery; it also would, by grouping critically ill patients in one place, relieve them of the need to travel hither and yon to change dressings and deliver daily care. With a hospital, a doctor could check on several patients in a short time, thus freeing him for other duties or more patients. If the new Annapolis Emergency Hospital proved well run, suitably equipped and staffed with good nurses, both the doctors and their patients would benefit. The doctors needed the hospital.

And the hospital needed the doctors—not only for their professional capabilities but because the paying patients they brought to the institution would offset the expense of serving those who could not pay. It was always the intent of the Annapolis Emergency Hospital Association to provide the hospital's services to all who needed them, regardless of financial status.

Through the spring and early summer of 1902, the Board of Managers worked to turn the old residence into a modern hospital. Rooms were converted into two wards—one for white patients and one for black patients, with a total of nine beds—and two private rooms for paying patients. The operating room, organized and equipped under direction of the medical staff, received close attention. Gas lighting and a telephone were installed and Miss Kate Andrews presented the hospital with a silver tea service. Nellie M. Pusey, a trained nurse, was hired as nurse-superintendent, with a pupil nurse to assist her.

On July 18, 1902, the new Annapolis Emergency Hospital opened its doors to its first patient, Mr. J. M. Bowers, foreman of the cut stone workers on the new Court of Appeals building.

As the first few patients received treatment, renovations of the Seidewitz home continued. Windows were screened, the plumbing repaired and a morgue, called the Dead House or Peace Chamber, was planned for the southern corner of the property. The board accepted cast-off toilets from the State House but found them unsuitable and had to buy new ones. Residents of Glen Burnie gave the hospital a cow, which was stabled at Mrs. Sturdy's on Murray Avenue until the expense of keeping it outweighed the benefits and it was sold to Emma Gage in 1903.

A private room cost $12 a week, semi-private $8 and ward beds $5, with all meals, dressings and nursing care included. Visiting hours for wards were allowed on Wednesday, Friday and Sunday from 11 a.m. to 5 p.m. The nurses, orderly and servants lived in the hospital.

By December 1, 1902, when the Annapolis Emergency Hospital Association held its first annual meeting, the hospital had treated 47

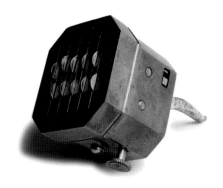

cases, eight of which were surgical. Dr. W. Clement Claude, chief of staff, reported that prospective patients had often been refused because of overcrowding. Miss Pusey and the pupil nurse had worked with scant rest or recreation. The types of cases listed by Dr. Claude suggest the nature of the hospital's services that first year. Of the 34 diagnoses, at least 19 were wounds or injuries: lacerations (four), broken bones (four), a gunshot wound, a dislocated shoulder, a concussion. Medical patients included three with typhoid fever, two with tuberculosis and "La Grippe," and one each with pneumonia and malaria. The operations performed included two appendectomies and three "excision of tumors." Five patients died: two with typhoid fever, one with tuberculosis, one with sarcoma and one with appendicitis. The latter, Charles Crawford, was the only surgical death. But, as Dr. Claude stated at the annual meeting of the association in 1902, "The apparent high rate of mortality is due to the fact that this is an emergency hospital only and almost every case so far received as a house patient has been of the utmost gravity."

The hospital's name and its purpose as a critical care facility were in accord with the thinking of the day. Before about 1890, most hospitals were found in urban areas and were designed for the treatment and/or housing of the poor, the chronically ill, the insane, the infectious, the aged—people without homes or resources. Dispensaries, or the outpatient clinics of these city hospitals, treated emergency patients who had no private physician. Isolation hospitals, often located on the outskirts of cities and towns, quarantined but usually did not cure victims of smallpox or cholera. Annapolis for years had had its own smallpox hospital, built in 1864 on the poorhouse lot along the

Annapolis and Elkridge Railroad behind the federal cemetery, on what is now Taylor Avenue. Dr. Dennis Claude Handy, a cousin of Dr. W. Clement Claude, received $100 a month for treating patients there in the late 1860s.

For most Americans, however, illness or injury was a responsibility of the home. The doctor would visit and nursing care might be provided by trained private duty nurses, but the patient remained in his accustomed surroundings and either improved or died.

The traditional municipal almshouse hospital of the 18th and 19th centuries, with its grim crowded wards and untrained nurses culled from the ranks of recovering patients, was not the sort of hospital founded in Annapolis in 1902, nor was it the sort of hospital being established elsewhere in rural Maryland at about the same time. In 1910, 10 hospitals in the counties of Maryland requested state aid. Six of them, in addition to the Annapolis Emergency Hospital, were acute care facilities opened between 1902 and 1907: Frederick City Hospital in Frederick (incorporated in 1898, but opened May 1, 1902), Washington County Hospital in Hagerstown (1905), Allegany Hospital in Cumberland (1905), Emergency Hospital in Easton (1906), Union Hospital in Elkton (1903) and General and Marine Hospital in Crisfield (1907). Allegany Hospital had no free beds and was the only applicant denied state aid. The rest, including the Annapolis Emergency Hospital and Peninsula General Hospital in Salisbury (founded in 1897), demonstrated the characteristics of the community hospital: they provided a mixture of free, paid and part-pay beds, were governed by a volunteer Board of Directors or Managers, were nonprofit and enjoyed the support of local individuals, businesses and civic groups.

The community hospital movement in America thrived in the decades before World War I. Almost all of these institutions relied financially on a combination of government funding, donations and private paying patients who were drawn to these new facilities because now, for the first time in the history of medicine, certain procedures could be accomplished better in a public institution than at home, no matter how luxurious or well staffed that home might be.

This is not to say that every American leaped at the opportunity to avail himself of his local hospital. The notion that "the hospital is where you go to die" remained strong even in the face of mortality statistics to the contrary. (The Annapolis Emergency Hospital rarely had an annual inpatient mortality rate above 4 percent.) Yet, as medical science developed, so did the community's sense that it was best practiced in a hospital.

The Annapolis Emergency Hospital Association finished out the year 1902 in the black by $168 out of a budget of $5,760, including the $3,500 purchase of the Seidewitz property and $1,266 to outfit the dwelling as a hospital. Salaries for 1902 totaled $400 and operating expenses, $361. The $215 received from paying patients amounted to only 28 percent of the maintenance costs, whereas membership in the association and dues equaled $1,645.

Despite its successful beginning, during the first full year of operation in 1903, the Annapolis Emergency Hospital came very close to failure. Rumors of a dispute between the Board of Managers and the medical staff and superintendent had appeared as early as September 27, 1902, when the *Baltimore World* hinted at incompetent surgery in the

death of Charles Crawford: "Now there is trouble among the board as they think the head nurse and local physicians are running things too much their way." Although the board dismissed this article as "yellow journalism," arguments among the medical staff, superintendent and board members increased as the months passed. At issue was the question of who controlled the hospital. The managers saw themselves as just that—managers. They assumed responsibility for the day-to-day operation of the hospital, the collection and disbursement of funds, the employment of nurses and servants, and the official appointment of the medical staff. Dr. Claude and the various members of the medical staff, however, believed that the physicians should and did have the right to direct the nurses and other employees, oversee the hospital's management and be provided with the equipment they believed necessary for the welfare of their patients.

Exacerbating this basic disagreement was the lack of funding sufficient to run the hospital, let alone improve the physical plant. The sewer installed by Mr. Seidewitz was inadequate, the plumbing leaked, the pipes froze. By April 1903, with expenditures averaging over $400 a month, the board found itself with only $600 in the treasury. Two benefit lectures and $100 from the Naval Academy chaplain helped only temporarily. When the board proposed firing the two pupil nurses and deferred the purchase of some surgical instruments, Dr. Claude protested strongly.

The issue came to a head over the employment of Nurse Pusey. The board asked for her resignation in March, saying that they were not satisfied with her management. When Miss Pusey, with the support of Drs. Claude and Welch, confronted the managers, the board just stood up and walked out of the hospital. The situation got worse over the next months. Nurse Pusey refused to leave the building on July 14 at the end of her year's contract, saying that neither she nor "her board" (the doctors) recognized the authority of the Board of Managers. Dr. Claude and others brought suit against the board to prohibit them from firing Miss Pusey. The board retaliated with a suit of its own. For four months Miss Pusey ran the hospital, using the money collected from paying patients for expenses. Finally, the courts having decided in favor of the Board of Managers, Dr. Claude gave the nurses a vacation and locked the hospital doors on October 1, 1903. The board reopened the building two days later with a new superintendent, Miss Ruth Adamson.

On December 7, 1903, some 600–800 men and women "of all creeds and all political connections" overflowed the Assembly

Nurses relax on the porch of the original Annapolis Emergency Hospital.

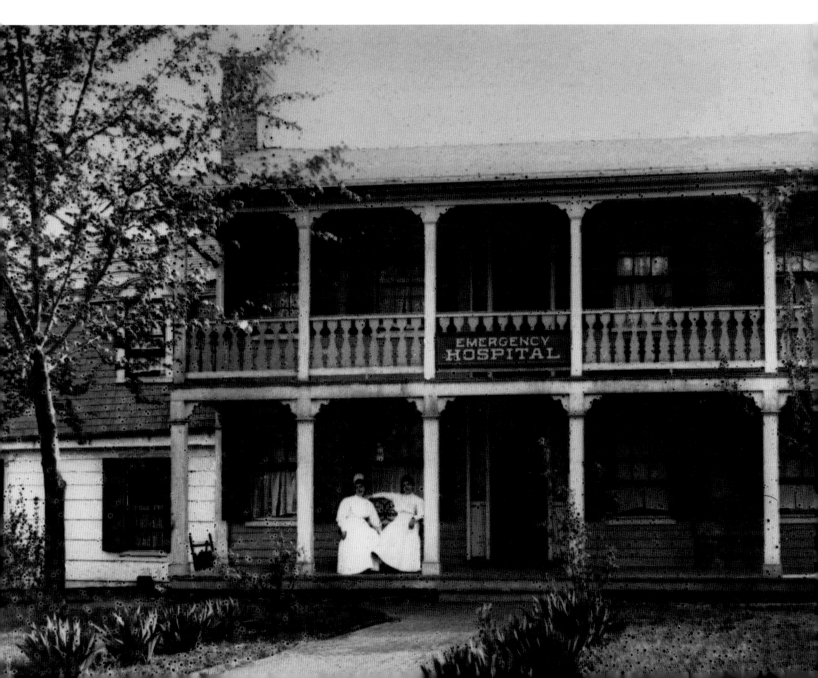

Rooms at City Hall for the second annual meeting of the Annapolis Emergency Hospital Association to vote for one of two proposed slates of officers: the ladies, both original members and new candidates, or the men, including Mayor DuBois and Drs. T. C. Walton and Frank H. Thompson. "Nothing has excited as much interest here ever before as this hospital controversy," claimed the *Evening Capital*, and the paper reported the outcome in its headlines:

WOMEN VICTORIOUS
Overwhelming Majority for the Board of
Lady Managers Over Men

EMERGENCY HOSPITAL ADMINISTRA-
TION ENDORSED BY PUBLIC
Men Turned Down and Entire Women's
Ticket Elected—
Board's Annual Report Approved—
Amendments Adopted

The ladies' slate was elected by a more than two-to-one majority. With the rulings of the court and a clear mandate from the people, the lady board would retain its power for 40 years. Elected to the board at this meeting was, among others, Kate Randall, one of the early members of the Hospital Club.

Even with the year's troubles, hospital admissions had climbed to 74, about three-quarters of whom were free patients, and hospital expenses totaled more than $3,700. The challenge of the lady board was clearly to raise more money. Again the managers approached the state for an increase in the appropriation and were awarded grants of $2,500 annually for the next two years. The city of Annapolis raised its funding to $200 a year.

Perhaps with second thoughts about their ability to manage or perhaps to placate those

who clearly thought they could not, the board amended its bylaws in 1904, setting up an advisory board of five men to "assist and advise the managers and audit the treasurer's accounts." Members of the first advisory board were Dr. George Wells, James M. Munroe, John dePeyster Douw, James P. Bannon and Robert J. Berryman.

The medical staff changed significantly in 1904. Drs. Claude, T. C. Walton, Frank H. Thompson and Sewell S. Hepburn resigned—not surprisingly, but not permanently. Dr. Bishop and another local physician, Dr. Elijah Williams, had died. They were replaced by Drs. J. S. Hayes and J. Oliver Purvis and the two Drs. Henkel: Charles B. and his nephew Louis B., Jr. Added to the consulting staff were surgeons St. Clair Spruill of the University of Maryland and Harvey Cushing of Johns Hopkins. The Annapolis and Baltimore Short Line Railroad gave passes to the consulting staff for their trips to and from Annapolis.

Improvements during 1904 included electric lighting and a new steam heating plant, with its boiler and pipes carefully covered with asbestos. At the close of the year, the board gave a grand three-day benefit bazaar at the Assembly Rooms. The event was opened by Governor Edwin Warfield, whose wife had recently been elected to the board. The more than $1,500 raised by the bazaar allowed the hospital to end the following year free of debt.

Confidence in the hospital may have waned in 1904, when only 50 patients sought care, but in 1905 the number rose to 219, of whom 79 were treated in the hospital and 140 used its dispensary services. There were 40 surgical cases and 39 medical cases. Even when the nurses and the orderly gave up their rooms to

A BOARD OF WOMEN MANAGERS [KNOW] ABOUT AS MUCH HOW TO CONDUCT A HOSPITAL AS 'CART DRIVERS'.

DR. W. CLEMENT CLAUDE, CHIEF OF STAFF
Evening Capital
December 7, 1903

allow 14 beds instead of 11, the hospital was pressed to accommodate the influx of patients. The installation of electric bells helped nurses cope and a larger sterilizer was added to the operating room.

Realizing that the hospital needed regular income beyond that provided by the state and local governments and ad hoc donations, no matter how generous, the board initiated two annual fundraisers for the weekend before Thanksgiving—Donation Day and Hospital Sunday. Money, supplies or food were welcomed, and these annual events contributed substantially to the hospital's income over the years.

By 1906, it seemed the new Annapolis Emergency Hospital had hit its stride. There were and would be yearly changes in the nursing and medical staffs, the advisory board and the lady managers, but Phoebe Martin, president of the board, with Emma Feldmeyer as treasurer and Kate Randall as secretary, seemed to have instituted routines that permitted the board and medical staff to work together. Each month, three members of the board were appointed as an executive committee to supervise and inspect the hospital on a daily basis.

Patients were admitted almost daily to the hospital—502 of them in 1906. The orderly had to move out of the hospital entirely during peak periods and the assistant nurses took turns using the room. The annual budget was close to $6,500, with paying patients contributing only about 17 percent of the income.

Both the board and the medical staff agreed that a larger, modern hospital was needed and that the financing would have to come from a source other than receipts and donations. Chief of Staff Dr. George Wells pro-posed at the annual meeting of the Annapolis Emergency Hospital Association in December 1906 that, since "all accident cases on the state's new building having been treated here at this hospital," the legislature should be asked for $25,000 to erect a new hospital at the front of the old building. A building fund was opened with the Annapolis Savings Institution.

Over the next two years, the number of patients continued to increase—to 610 in 1907 and 1,156 in 1908—and the cottage hospital strained at its seams. Private rooms were reserved months in advance and paying patients often had to be accommodated in wards.

The annual budget kept pace through the efforts of local citizens, who continued to hold fundraisers and contribute through their churches on Hospital Sundays. Businesses donated supplies. Robert J. Berryman, a member of the advisory board and president of the Annapolis Ice Manufacturing Company, for instance, provided the hospital with 25 pounds of ice each day for years.

Finally in 1909, the state raised its annual appropriation to $5,000 and authorized the requested $25,000 for a new building. Work began immediately on a three-story brick structure facing Franklin Street. During construction, the old cottage hospital continued its work, treating 1,001 cases in both the hospital and the dispensary in 1909. Of 101 surgical house patients and 23 medical patients, only six died.

By 1910, the years of the cottage hospital were at an end. In its first eight years, more than 3,600 patients had come through the doors of the Annapolis Emergency Hospital and most had found solace and healing there.

set up practice in July 1929 in south county. I had just worked for a year at Johns Hopkins in the clinic, but I'm a country girl so I thought I'd come down here to try it out.

I let people know I was setting up practice and sat in my office for a week before I finally got my first patient. A car pulled up front and two men got out. They had a big collie dog with a gash in its head. I sewed the gash up, and that was my first patient!

In those days there were only two paved roads in the county. If you needed to see patients in the winter, you rode horseback or walked to their home. I saw sick people, delivered babies and even did an emergency appendectomy one time.

Most days I saw patients in my office in the morning, then went to the hospital to see my patients there. Then I'd go to patients' homes in the afternoon. Sometimes patients would come to my home at night. I got to be close friends with many patients. I charged $1 for an office visit, $4 for a home visit and $15 to deliver a baby. I sure didn't get rich and most of the time I didn't get paid anything.

When I couldn't solve something at home, I sent patients to the hospital. You can imagine it could be tough to get up there. At first they told me, 'You can't be a member of the hospital staff. You live too far away!'

Things were pretty basic at the hospital, but they did the best they could with what they had. There were two wards downstairs and a few patient rooms upstairs. I spent the night curled up at the bottom of a good many patients' beds. The sickest patients went up to Hopkins, but going to Baltimore was like going to China.

It was a good life. I enjoyed it; it's what I always wanted to do. And the hospital just grew like anything.

Perspective...

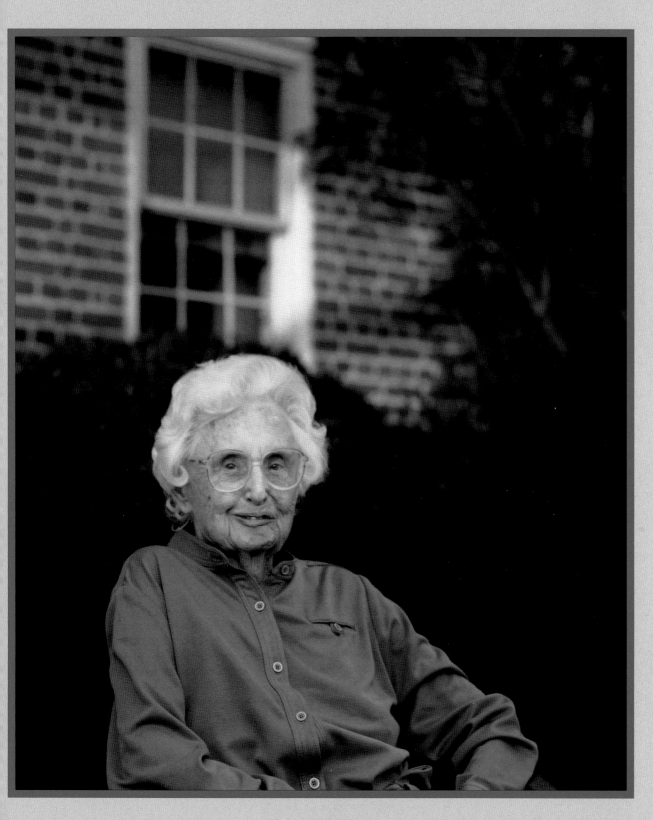

Dr. Emily Wilson

Born in South Carolina, 1904

First female physician in southern Anne Arundel county, 1929

Medical staff president, 1953

The managers devoted most of their energies during 1910 to furnishing the new hospital building on Franklin Street. Constructed with a state appropriation of $25,000 in 1909 and additional funds donated by civic organizations and individuals, the building was opened for public inspection in early December 1910.

Harry J. Hopkins, chief clerk in the State Comptroller's Office and later president of Farmers National Bank, was treasurer of the building committee as well as a longtime member of the hospital's advisory board. Other members of the building committee were Dr. George Wells, the chief of staff; Dr. Walton H. Hopkins, Dr. William S. Welch and Dr. J. Oliver Purvis of the medical staff; A. Theodore Brady, state delegate (1908) and senator (1910) from Anne Arundel County; and Judge James R. Brashears of the Circuit Court.

The new hospital, with its three-story center block and two-story wings on either side, contained operating rooms, three wards of six beds each, a small three-bed ward for children and nine private rooms, as well as rooms for the superintendent and nurses, a new kitchen, heating plant, laundry and parlor. Private rooms were furnished at about $100 each by the Odd Fellows, Redmen, Elks, Masons and by private individuals, including Mrs. Williard Brownson, wife of a former Naval Academy superintendent, and Misses Margaret and Blanche Martin. The furniture in rooms previously maintained by the Peggy Stewart Tea Party chapter of the Daughters of the American Revolution and Mrs. John Schouler, wife of Adm. John Schouler, was moved to the new building. (Mrs. Curtis J. Nice had also furnished a room in the old hospital as a memorial to her husband, Dr. Nice.) Fees for private rooms were set at

$12–$15 per week for those on the second floor and $8–$10 for those on the third floor. While the operating rooms were equipped under the direction of the medical staff, the board pored over catalogs and ventured out to Philadelphia and Baltimore to inspect first-hand the beds (iron), mattresses, hair and feather pillows, and other furniture necessary for the new rooms. They purchased kitchen equipment, including a new coal-fired range and a "large improved coffee machine." The three assistant nurses were set to work cutting and binding new blankets. Miss Kate Randall, board secretary, began the Children's Hospital Club, whose members contributed a penny a week toward the furnishing of the children's ward. By year's end, 220 members had collected $18. The ladies of the Chase Home made dozens of caps and stockings for the operating room. Shortly before the official opening in December, the board engaged carpenters to install closets for the nurses' rooms, which the architects evidently deemed "unnecessary luxuries."

Finally, on December 3 and 4, the patients were moved to the new building. Just before the annual meeting of the Annapolis Emergency Hospital Association on Monday, December 5, the hospital was dedicated in ceremonies led by Rev. Joseph P. McComas of St. Anne's and Rev. Walter G. McNeill of the First Methodist Episcopal Church.

The new hospital opened with a typhoid fever patient. He was the first of many cases admitted to the Annapolis Emergency Hospital over the next eight or nine months as Annapolis and the Naval Academy tried to cope with an outbreak of the dreaded disease. A result primarily of poor sanitation, which allowed the introduction of fecal matter into water or foods,

ANNAPOLIS HAS A REAL HOSPITAL *1910 - 1927*

typhoid fever (salmonella typhosa) surfaced periodically in Annapolis from the 18th to the early 20th century. Until the advent of antibiotics, treatment was limited to the relief of symptoms and good nursing care. If the contamination was a single source and the infected persons were isolated immediately, the disease could be kept under control. If, on the other hand, the source was a public well or reservoir, epidemics were not uncommon.

In the 1910–11 outbreak, the culprits were found to be an old well in the Germantown area and, for the Naval Academy, contaminated milk. More than 200 midshipmen were vaccinated with antityphoid serum. Annapolitans were cautioned against using public drinking cups and roller towels. Cases continued to appear throughout the spring and early summer, and Dr. John T. Russell of Eastport, a physician on the medical staff, was among those spending several weeks in the hospital. In July, when local residents complained of a peculiar taste and smell to the city's water, Dr. J. J. Murphy, then chief of staff, reassured them that the water from the city's drought-depleted reservoir, while disagreeable, was probably not dangerous. He

Annapolis Emergency Hospital, c.1910.

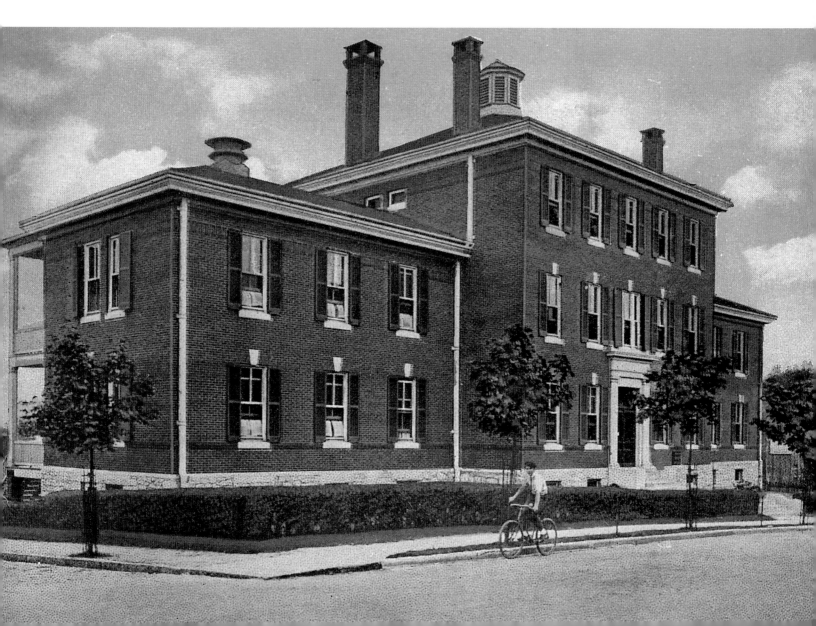

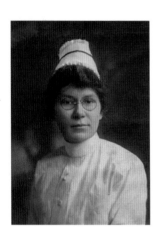

advised boiling it just in case. Although the midshipmen survived the fever without loss of life, a number of townspeople died. The hospital's statistics for 1910 showed a total of 22 deaths out of the 300 cases admitted to the hospital. Nine of these deaths resulted from the year's 422 surgical procedures, but the unusually high death rate of 7.3 percent included a large number of medical deaths, presumably because of the typhoid epidemic. More than 2,000 patients were treated at the dispensary that year.

According to Charles Rosenberg, there were, in 1880, only 15 nursing schools in the country with perhaps 300 graduates. Thirty years later the situation was quite different. Large hospitals such as Johns Hopkins established nurse training schools in conjunction with medical schools. But it was the community hospital movement of the early 20th century that made nursing careers possible for thousands of young women. The benefits were mutual and obvious. Hospitals, especially community-supported hospitals in small towns, were in chronic financial trouble. Students provided them with a fairly constant, inexpensive supply of suitable young women eager to learn good nursing skills and practice them on the hospital's patients. For the prospective nurse, timid of big city life but desirous of achieving her chosen profession, her local community hospital offered an attractive alternative.

As the board and medical staff discussed plans for the new Annapolis Emergency Hospital in the fall of 1910, the staffing demands of the larger building led them to consider implementing a training school of their own. Three of the staff physicians offered to teach classes, and Miss Rosamond Minnis, the loyal and conscientious superintendent, agreed to direct the students.

On April 20, 1911, incorporation papers for the Annapolis Emergency Hospital Training School for Nurses were signed. The incorporation was a joint effort of the medical staff: Drs. James J. Murphy, William S. Welch, Oscar H. McNamara, J. Oliver Purvis, Walton H. Hopkins and John T. Russell; and the Board of Managers, represented by Eleanor R. Dashiell, Emma N. Feldmeyer, Julia M. Tisdale, Kate D. Andrews, Kate W. Randall and Phoebe E. Martin. The first three students were accepted in February 1911.

Student nurses were required to be single, of good character and to have had sufficient education to enable them to master the rigorous course work. The curriculum of the school included anatomy and physiology, *materia medica*, general medicine, bacteriology, bandaging, hygiene and sanitation, and practical nursing in the first year; intermediate anatomy and physiology and *materia medica*, gynecology, "urianalysis," obstetrics and practical nursing during the second year; and diseases of children, general surgery, anesthetics, nervous and mental diseases, dietetics and more practical nursing for the third year, or senior, nurses. By 1914, Dr. Purvis was in charge of the program.

The students lived in the hospital under the supervision of the head nurse-superintendent. When they were not in class, they gained their practical nursing experience on the floor caring for patients. Recreation was limited; hours were long. At the completion of their training in Annapolis, graduate nurses took a state board examination. In 1915, the Annapolis Emergency Hospital nurses received the second highest average score of nurses from all the schools in the state taking the exam.

Ida Rose White, who entered the training

BOIL ALL THE DRINKING WATER! SWAT ALL THE FLIES!

DR. J. J. MURPHY, CHIEF OF STAFF
Evening Capital
July 31, 1911
In response to the typhoid fever epidemic

school at age 17 on February 28, 1911, was the school's first graduate at exercises held at the hospital on December 1, 1913. Decorated for Christmas with holly and red-shaded lights, the hospital sun parlor was filled with the sound of violin and cello, played by members of the Naval Academy band. In attendance for the special occasion were Mayor James F. Strange, the town's clergy, all of the physicians of the hospital and the Board of Managers. Chief of Staff Dr. J. J. Murphy presented Miss White with her diploma; the Hon. James M. Munroe delivered the major address of the evening. After the ceremonies, the nurses held a dance in the first floor women's ward, "cleared for the occasion," and enjoyed refreshments in the nurses' dining room. In later years, the graduation and the traditional dance were held in the Assembly Rooms of City Hall or in the St. John's College gymnasium.

Medical workers are subject to two special perils: they can sicken and die from diseases contracted from their patients and, especially in a community hospital, their dying patients may be close friends. Nursing students in the early days of the Annapolis Emergency Hospital learned these lessons along with anatomy and *materia medica.* Nursing records show several students as "transferring to Sabillasville." Sabillasville, in northern Frederick County, was the location of a state tuberculosis sanatorium. Whether these transfers were the result of a better job offer or infection with the disease itself is not always clear, but in at least one case, there is a note: "died T.B."

And then there was the experience of Lillian Mae Simmons. In the spring of 1918, she was in her last year at the hospital's nursing school and engaged to be married to Tommy Mullaney, a 21-year-old ironworker from New York who had come to Annapolis to work on the first radio towers built at North Severn. At noon on April 23, 1918, Mullaney fell 300 feet from his tower. His friends rushed him to the Annapolis Emergency Hospital, but at 12:30 p.m. Dr. Sewell Hepburn pronounced him dead of a fractured skull. Miss Simmons, on duty at the time, collapsed in anguish. Her mother was pregnant with her 13th child at the time; when the daughter was born in August, she was named Helen Mullaney after Tommy Mullaney's sister.

Dr. Frances Edith Weitzman joined the medical staff of the Annapolis Emergency Hospital in 1912 as its first woman physician. In 1915, when Margaret Wohlgemuth became superintendent and director of the nurses' training program at the Annapolis Emergency Hospital, she and Dr. Weitzman organized the hospital's first maternity ward. Before then, only a few critically ill maternity patients had been admitted. Six babies were born in the hospital that first year and, in 1916, when the hospital reported 35 births, the ladies of the community began serious fundraising for a maternity ward. Three years later, in January 1919, a six-patient maternity ward was opened, with a fully equipped delivery room and a nursery for eight infants. In 1920, 106 babies were born at the Annapolis Emergency Hospital and maternity patients became an important source of revenue for the hospital. Having all their patients in one place was a boon to the attending physicians and, for expectant mothers, the availability of appropriate surgical backup made hospital deliveries attractive.

In addition to the need for maternity care, the advantages of an isolation ward became apparent in 1916 when several children contracted infantile paralysis (poliomyelitis). Two years later, the 1918 influenza epidemic threw

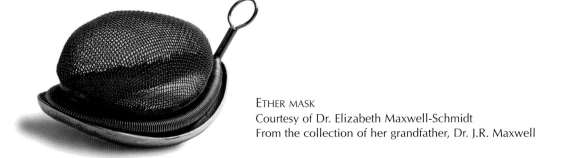

the hospital into a crisis. The epidemic began in Annapolis in early fall, just as three doctors on the staff left town for war-time duty. Drs. Walton H. Hopkins, J. Oliver Purvis and Frances E. Weitzman had accepted commissions in the army. Miss Margaret Wohlgemuth had volunteered in 1917 and was in Europe.

By late September 1918, the epidemic canceled public events. A curfew was instituted for children under 16 and the midshipmen were restricted to base. The hospital quickly filled with patients. With the help of orderlies loaned by the academy and women of the town who volunteered their services, Navy and local doctors and nurses worked day and night to relieve the suffering. On Sunday, October 13, at the height of the epidemic, churches remained closed. The silence of that morning, when for the first time in memory no Sunday bells rang, underscored the distress of the townspeople. There are no firm statistics on the number of influenza deaths in Anne Arundel County, but oral tradition indicates that they were considerable. At least one nurse at the hospital died.

By late October, the epidemic had abated. Midshipmen again received town liberty and the hospital board turned once more to financial problems.

Equipping and furnishing the new hospital in 1910 and 1911, at a cost greater than the board had planned, initiated a period of deficit spending. The board borrowed from Farmers National Bank and, in the years that followed, when city and state appropriations came in later than expected, it was forced to borrow again. Concurrent with these difficulties was a change in attitude that increased demands on the building's facilities: when people got sick, they sought hospital care rather than home care. The number of patients in maternity, children's and isolation wards increased, and the nurses' training school would require separate housing for students if it were to continue to grow.

The hospital's finances depended on paying patients and the services of the student nurses; its mission was to provide proper accommodations and treatment for all those who were sick. The physical plant needed to be enlarged.

In the spring of 1918, Edwin Seidewitz offered the hospital board the rest of his property between Franklin Street, Cathedral Street, the land of James W. Murray to the south and the creek. W. Meade Holladay, publisher of the *Anne Arundel Advertiser* and a member of the hospital's advisory board, took an option on the property for $9,000, pledged $100 himself and initiated a community drive to raise the rest. A $5,000 mortgage on the lot could be continued; the board would need $4,000 to make the purchase. The community responded enthusiastically and by late June the money had been secured. The transfer from Seidewitz to the Annapolis Emergency Hospital Association, dated May 21, 1918, enlarged the hospital's grounds to 310 feet along Franklin Street and about 320 feet on Cathedral. Neither Shaw nor the lower part of South Street were cut through and the creek still bulged up into the lower section of the hospital land. In about 1923, a bulkhead was built from the foot of Charles Street across Acton Cove and the land side filled in with trash, debris and dirt. Shaw and South streets were completed by 1930.

Far from being able to begin construction on new buildings in 1918 and 1919, the hospital had trouble just keeping itself in business. The fact that hospital debt was widespread throughout Maryland at this time did not help. Demands by the hospital workers for salary increases, the loss of staff doctors to the war effort, the tremendous pressure imposed on the facilities and staff by the influenza epidemic, and a decrease in state funding all placed the Annapolis hospital in serious financial straits. Money for annual maintenance had to be assured before capital improvements could be considered. The annual budget at that time was more than $25,000.

Again the hospital turned to the community. In September 1919, both the Eastport and Rescue Hose volunteer fire companies donated portions of their carnival proceeds to the hospital. The following month the Annapolis Emergency Hospital Association launched a drive for annual memberships, which it hoped would provide a sustained permanent income. A house-to-house canvas throughout Annapolis and the county ensued, with volunteers calling on all families, black and white, to make five-year pledges to the hospital. Results of the drive were disappointing; by November only about $4,500 had been raised in pledges and gifts. One of those gifts was $26.15, the proceeds of a spelling bee at St. Margaret's Hall.

Nevertheless, the 1919 annual report showed almost $17,000 received in donations during the year. State, county and city appropriations totaled less than $6,500. Expenses were $28,531, but the balance on hand at the end of the year was almost $8,500. Considering that the balance from 1918's receipts had been only $58, the hospital's financial picture had improved significantly.

The year 1919 brought a number of changes to the hospital and its staff. In July, Emma Feldmeyer retired after 15 years as treasurer of the association. From 1905, when she took over the books, until 1919, the yearly cost of maintaining the hospital had risen from $4,268 to more than $28,000. She had been praised routinely by the auditing committee of the advisory board for her meticulous bookkeeping, her efficiency and her accuracy. To Mrs. Feldmeyer, Phoebe Martin, who retired in 1916 after 11 years as board president, Kate Randall, the secretary from 1905 until her death in 1922, and Kate Andrews, secretary and later president of the board, is due much of the credit for the early success of the hospital. Membership on the board was a natural outlet for women of managerial or leadership ability whose sex and social position precluded them from remunerative employment.

Also in 1919, Superintendent Margaret Wohlgemuth's return pleased everyone. She was a local woman, well liked, and her resumption of duties at the Annapolis Emergency Hospital was heralded by an article and photograph in the *Evening Capital*, which called her a woman "of marked executive ability and wide experience in nursing."

In September 1919, the hospital established a U.S. Venereal Clinic in the basement under the direction of Dr. Purvis. Patients were treated free of charge under a program sponsored by the federal government and the Maryland Board of Health.

The hospital's first radiology department opened in 1919 with one X-ray machine and the services of Dr. L. P. O'Donnell, "an expert Roentgenologist." Dr. O'Donnell was on duty in the hospital for three hours each day and on call at other times. X-rays had been introduced for hospital use in 1896 and their capabilities as an aid to diagnosis made them

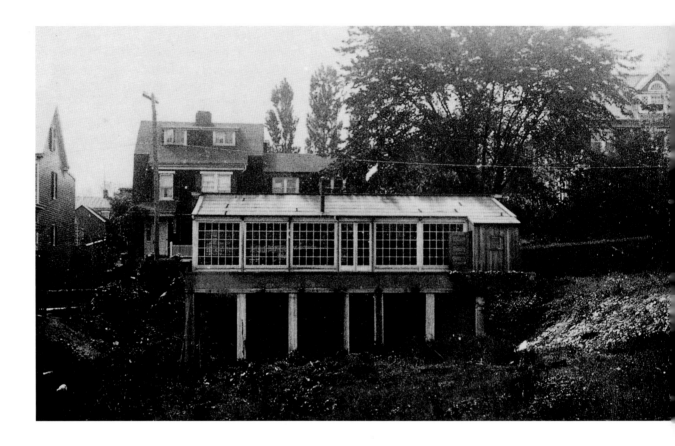

popular immediately, although their expense and the need for a trained operator kept them out of community hospitals for some years. The Annapolis Emergency Hospital was very proud of its new machine and 200 patients were X-rayed during its first year of service. By 1924, the department collected $25,000 a year, of which half went to the hospital, and in 1925 a filing cabinet was purchased and films arranged numerically. Navy doctors often served as radiologists for the Annapolis Emergency Hospital.

Finally in 1920, the Annapolis Emergency Hospital board and staff saw the realization of the long-awaited Nurses' Home. Built on a 50-foot lot on Franklin Street just south of the hospital, it was completed late in the year. Furnishing the building and making it ready for occupancy became the focus of a new organization, the hospital Auxiliary, founded by Mrs. D. N. Carpenter, wife of a doctor at the Naval Academy. Dr. Carpenter was elected treasurer and Henry F. Sturdy, a professor at the academy, became the group's first secretary and, later, its president.

With the stated purpose to raise funds for the hospital, especially for the Nurses' Home, the hospital Auxiliary reached out into the community, setting up "departments," or branches, of the Auxiliary. By January 1921, 1,911 subscribers had contributed more than $7,000 in sums ranging from $1,000 to 50 cents. Auxiliary Department Number Two, "the colored Auxiliary," organized by Norman D. Cully, secured some 500 subscribers and received special praise for its efforts.

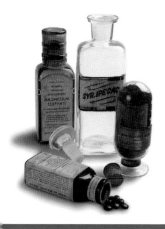

COLLECTION OF MEDICINES AND BOTTLES
Courtesy of AAMC Pharmacy

The Auxiliary paid for hospital awnings in 1923, as well as contributing $200 to the Nurses' Home. It also printed 1,000 jar labels for the pantry. Within the next few years, however, the Auxiliary's efforts died out, probably when Professor Sturdy, its staunchest supporter, was elected to the hospital's advisory board.

Shortly after purchasing the remaining Seidewitz property in 1918, the board sold the land farthest from the hospital—100 feet on Franklin Street back to the creek—to St. Anne's Church. Truxtun Beale acquired this land in 1920 and reconveyed it to the hospital along with a sun parlor, then under construction. The new building, completed in 1921, was mostly glass and resembled the greenhouses that had once stood nearby. Fresh air and sunshine were considered important to good health, and in an era when hospital stays might stretch into weeks, this new building was especially welcome. For the rest of its life, it was called the Glass House. Beale, an author and diplomat, owned Decatur House in Washington, D.C., and several large tracts of land in Anne Arundel County. Primrose Hill, just outside of Annapolis, was his country home.

The Children's Hospital Club, begun in 1910 by Kate Randall, continued its good work and in 1921 entirely refurnished the children's ward—proving what can come of saving a penny a week, as the children of Annapolis did for so long. For years the children paid for the entire cost of maintaining the children's ward.

Beds and rooms and even the operating room became apt memorials to beloved family members and most were marked with appropriate plaques. Donation Days and Hospital Sundays afforded even the poorest citizens

the opportunity to support the work of the hospital. But money was not the only kind of gift bestowed upon this institution by the people of Annapolis and Anne Arundel County. Every month the hospital received gifts of canned goods, sugar, meats, vegetables, cakes (often for the nurses), eggs, rabbits, preserves, buttermilk, magazines and daily newspapers, spring water, poultry, toys for the children, fruits (sometimes shipped from Florida) and handmade baby clothes. The donors were ladies of Annapolis, Eastport, and the county, schools, civic groups, Sunday school classes and businesses. During the month of December 1922 alone, the nurses received seven-and-a-half cakes, three of them fruitcakes.

The hospital's first clinical laboratory opened in January 1922. Paying patients remaining in the hospital more than 24 hours were charged an additional fee of $1.50 for lab tests. One of the senior nurses took a special course at the University of Maryland and was placed in charge under the direction of Dr. Purvis, chief of staff. In 1925, the lab was fully equipped and a trained technician took over.

Governor Albert Ritchie attended the annual meeting of the Annapolis Emergency Hospital Association on October 16, 1922, to hear Miss Kate Andrews, board president, announce that the hospital debt had been "entirely wiped out" and that plans were being made to enlarge the third floor of the hospital. The Naval Academy Chapel contributed the first $100 toward the new building fund and academy children donated to the new maternity ward, which was the focus of the board's plans for renovation. A special naval committee was organized under Mrs. Thomas R. Kurtz, wife of the academy's commandant.

The hospital housed 946 patients in 1923, 139

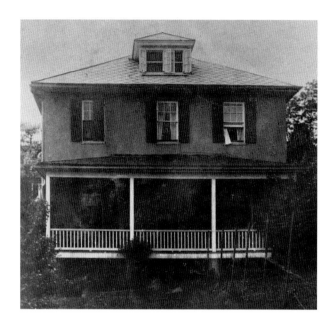

of them obstetrical cases, and treated 917 patients from the dispensary. There appeared to be no doubt in anyone's mind that the building on Franklin Street needed to be bigger.

Before resigning as superintendent in October 1923, Miss Margaret Wohlgemuth reiterated the critical necessity for an isolation ward. Infectious patients menaced especially the surgical and obstetrical cases, she said, and put the hospital at risk.

The average hospital stay in 1924 was 11 days; medical cases numbered 282 and surgical cases 472; 42 in-house patients—4.7 percent—died. The operations performed that year included 38 appendectomies, 35 laparotomies, six caesareans and 132 nose and throat procedures. Disbursements for the year totaled more than $48,800.

The Woman's Club of Davidsonville painted five rooms. The hospital in 1925 repainted the Nurses' Home. Col. John A. Lockwood placed two electric lamps at the Franklin Street entrance of the hospital in memory of his niece, Miss Mary Louise Booth, in 1924. These lamps provided the inspiration for the hospital's logo.

A children's welfare clinic for white and black children was established in 1924, and a tuberculosis clinic, meeting weekly, began in 1925. Also in 1925, the board hired a trained dietitian to oversee patient's meals and teach the course in hospital dietetics to the student nurses.

The nursing staff in the mid-1920s consisted of the superintendent, an assistant superintendent who was in charge of the operating room, a graduate nurse for the second floor, a night superintendent, the dietitian and a graduate nurse/technician to give anesthesia. The nursing school had 12–14 students during the 1920s and graduated two or three nurses a year.

The operating rooms were painted and retiled in 1925 and an electric cautery and suction apparatus was installed. Mrs. Martin Smith donated a self-filling syringe for local anesthesia. The ward for black patients was redecorated with funds received from the black residents of the city and county for that purpose. Residents of Skidmore, led by Lizzie Smith, sold jumpers to contribute $40.

In 1926, the idea of enlarging the hospital had grown from just extending the third floor to building a new wing. With more than 1,000 in-house and 1,500 dispensary patients that year, only a substantial building program would serve the hospital's purposes. Professor Henry Sturdy, now a member of the advisory board, led the fight for the new annex.

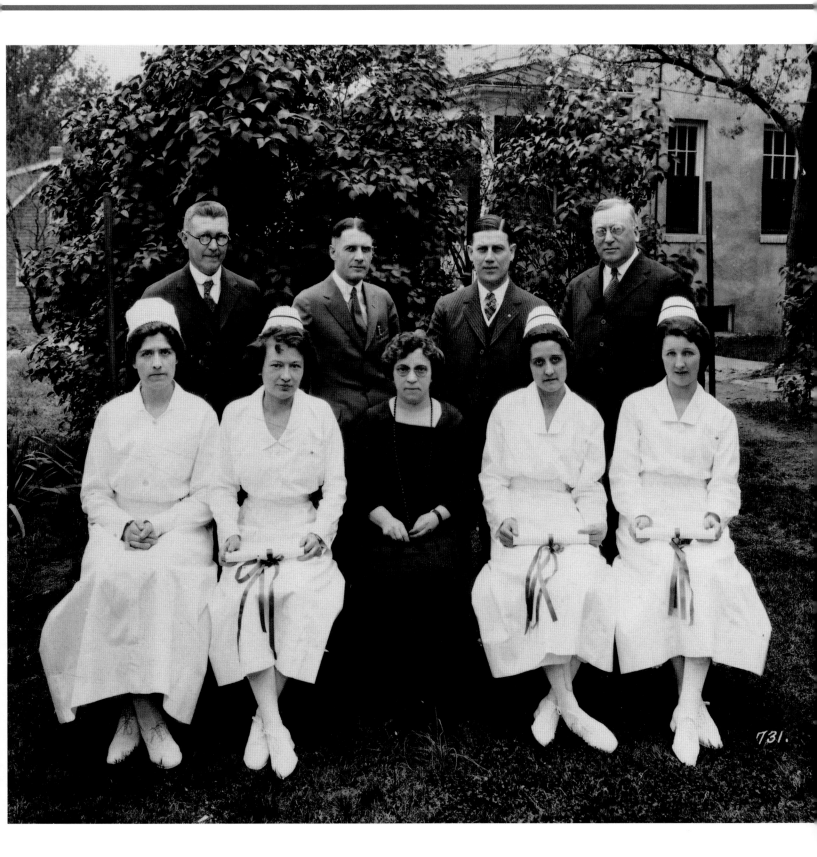

At the 25th annual meeting of the Annapolis Emergency Hospital Association in October 1927, President Kate Andrews announced the selection of Henry Powell Hopkins (son of Harry J. Hopkins, longtime member of the advisory board) and Allen Burton as architects of the annex, and of Mr. Sylvester Labrot as chairman of the building committee campaign. The state appropriated $40,000 of the estimated $100,000 cost of the new building. A building committee of board members, doctors, citizens and a member of the advisory board had, with the architects, planned the annex and submitted plans and specifications for bid.

The annex, 92 feet by 42 feet and facing Cathedral Street, would add 48 beds, including 19 beds for maternity patients, to the capacity of the hospital, as well as a multi-room dispensary, isolation room for ward patients, new heating plant, kitchen and service rooms.

Shortly after 3 a.m. on the cold, drizzly morning of Friday, December 16, 1927, Miss Marcellana Dulaney, the night superintendent, smelled smoke. She called Annapolis Fire Marshall Jesse Fisher and set about rousing the other nurses. Quickly they tagged the seven babies in the nursery and bundled them and their mothers out of the building. The youngest baby was just two days old. They and the other patients were handed over to the care of neighbors, who took them into their homes.

Marshall Fisher found the source of the fire in a storage room on the top floor; within minutes the flames spread through the rafters. Volunteer companies from the city, Eastport and West Annapolis responded. Fighting the fire from both the interior and exterior of the building, they battled smoke and heat and falling debris to save as much of the building as possible. Several fire fighters fell in the darkness or were overcome by smoke. Walter Scherger, a 26-year-old master carpenter at the Naval Academy and volunteer fireman, found a body in a third-floor bed amidst smoke and flames. Risking death, he grabbed the body and rushed with it to safety, only to discover he held a wax and straw dummy used by the nurses' school. The dietitian and two student nurses asleep on the third floor near the blaze escaped, but lost all their possessions.

Doctors from the town and the Naval Academy treated fire fighters and looked after the patients. Assisting them were Red Cross nurse Mrs. Sara Sutherland Green, formerly a nurse at the hospital, and Mayor Charles W. Smith. Local residents brought coffee to the firemen and comforted the sick.

Miraculously, all of the firemen and the 35 or so patients survived the fire, although Anthony Ayers, one of the most seriously ill at the time, died the following Monday. A few patients were taken to the Naval Academy hospital, but most returned to their homes and the hospital nurses visited them there.

The top floor of the main building and the wing at the corner of Franklin and Cathedral streets were the most heavily damaged; the other floors and the south wing suffered serious smoke and water damage. Some of the furnishings on the lower floors were saved, but the operating room and its equipment were destroyed. Insurance would cover most of the loss, but not any improvements.

The managers and medical staff met almost as soon as the fire was out to assess the damages and get the hospital back in business. The

Nurses' Home became a temporary hospital, the nurses moved to private homes and the women of Annapolis immediately began sewing and making bandages to replace the supplies lost in the fire.

Mr. Sylvester Labrot enlarged his fundraising goal to $100,000 to include an additional $40,000 to restore the old building. Among the early and significant contributors was the Guy Carleton Parlett Post No. 7 of the American Legion, which offered more than $4,000 set aside for a new Legion post, as a memorial to the soldiers, sailors and marines of Annapolis who served in World War I. The post's Auxiliary donated $275 to furnish a room in the new annex.

Within a week of the fire, almost $16,500, in amounts ranging from $5,000 (three) to 25 cents, was deposited in the building fund. Card parties (the Catholic Daughters, the DAR), dances (the Knights of Pythias) and other events were planned by civic groups. Contributions poured in from doctors, lodges, academy personnel, children and residents. The *Evening Capital* published the names of donors with the amount received and carried a daily front-page plea for more.

At the end of the its 25th year of service, there appeared to be no question in the community that the Annapolis Emergency Hospital was of tremendous importance to the health and well-being of Annapolis and the county.

Twenty-six-year-old Charles Wallace Hambrock watched the Annapolis Emergency Hospital burn from his parents' home on Franklin Street on December 16, 1927. Later, he created this painting from memory. It has graced the walls of the West Annapolis Volunteer Fire Department for over 60 years.

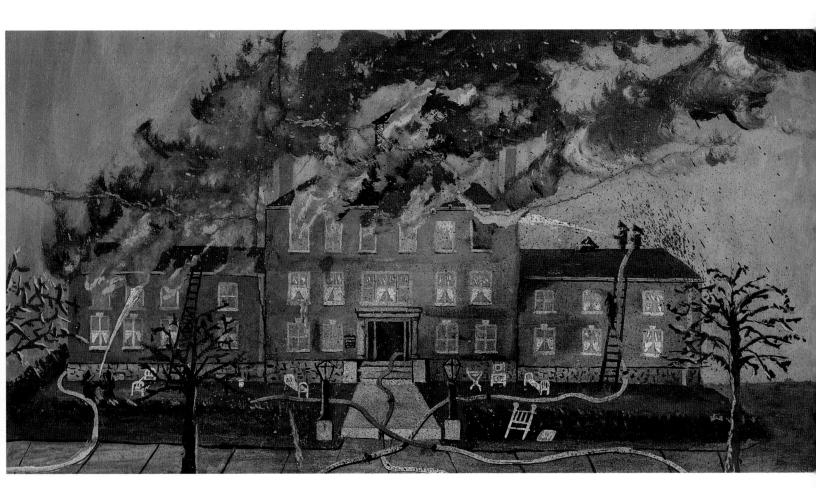

Annapolis residents always have been willing to help at the hospital.

I remember sometime in the late 1930s, four men were burned and they were in the hospital. They could not feed themselves, and the nurses didn't have time. There was no one to take care of them, so volunteers went in and helped out. That's the kind of cooperation there was between the hospital and the local residents.

We had a fundraiser around 1940 to raise money to help with the new building. Becky Clatanoff was heading it; they had a professional fundraiser come in but Becky arranged everything. She formed teams and assigned people to go see residents. You weren't calling on your friends, so that made it easier to ask for money. Most people were very generous. In fact you had to be careful that people weren't pledging more than they could give!

Out of that effort, the Auxiliary grew in 1944. It started out very small, but grew rapidly. People especially wanted to help with the hospital, because it was so important.

Auxiliary members started out fixing flowers for patients, because florists didn't send flowers that were already in arrangements. There was a book cart, too, donated by a local gentleman, and they would only accept hardbound books. While the new building was under construction, Auxiliary members would feed workers hot coffee when they came to work in the morning.

The Clothes Box was started in 1952. Two local ladies had started the business and they moved away. It was a nice little money-making thing, so they took it to the hospital administration and offered it to them. The administration turned it over to the Auxiliary. It grew by leaps and bounds.

The hospital has always occupied a soft spot in everyone's heart. Everyone wants to help. It's a part of Annapolis; it's always there. People have a feeling of confidence in the place; you feel safe.

Perspective...

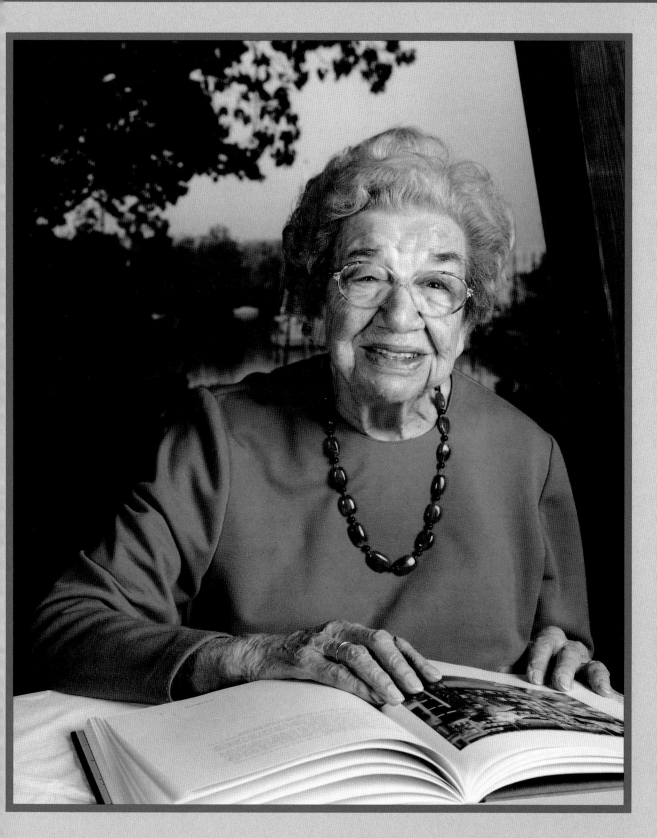

Bee Hiltabidle

Moved to Annapolis,
1937

Joined Auxiliary, 1950

Auxiliary president,
1952

Mother of Dr. Stephen
Hiltabidle, retired
AAMC surgeon

For nine months of 1928 following the fire, the Nurses' Home was pressed into service as a makeshift hospital. The Naval Academy hospital admitted and operated on emergency cases beyond the scope of the temporary building, sterilized dressings and took X-rays for the Annapolis physicians. Throughout that year, the citizens of Annapolis and Anne Arundel County—white and black, rich and poor—contributed money and assistance to restore their hospital, but the building committee's target of $100,000 for restoration of the old building and construction of the annex proved too much. Gifts from individuals, organizations and businesses totaled just over $64,000 by October.

Nevertheless, repairs to the damaged main building and construction of the annex began almost immediately after the fire. The architects, Hopkins and Burton, amended their plans and specifications, and Bean Brothers of Annapolis was awarded the construction

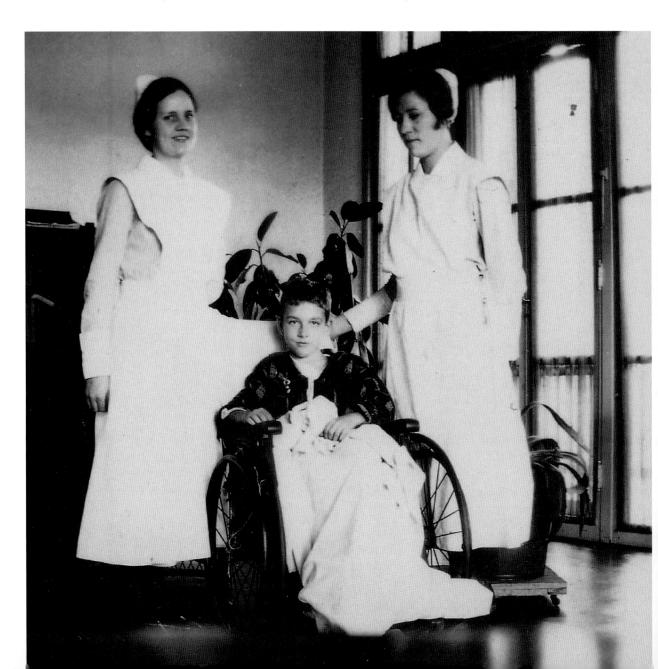

Patients and student nurses enjoyed the hospital's sun parlor.

EXPANSION UNDER THE LADY BOARD *1927 - 1944*

contract. The renovated main building opened for public inspection on September 6, 1928, and 15 patients were transferred from the Nurses' Home the next day. Only a few days later, a typhoid epidemic in Eastport hospitalized nine patients. Annapolis Emergency Hospital was back in business.

With all its problems, the hospital treated 886 in-house patients from October 1927 to October 1928. The renovated main building could accommodate 42 patients, with another 50 beds planned for the annex.

The interior of the original brick building was, to all intents and purposes, completely new. There were new floors, a new steel stairway and fire escapes, new plumbing, and a new elevator and shaft. The doorways were made large enough to roll a bed through and the interior walls and ceilings were freshly plastered and painted. The operating and sterilizing rooms received modern equipment and a new X-ray machine was purchased. The new heating plant was capable of heating the entire hospital and the Nurses' Home.

The long-awaited annex, redesigned to be completely fireproof, was built but only partially finished inside. The new kitchen and dining rooms and X-ray department in the basement were completed, but the upper floors, including the enlarged maternity ward and new dispensary, were left bare, pending additional funds. Even with this, the building committee reported a deficit of more than $20,000 at the October 1928 annual meeting.

Some nurses in training took classes at the University of Maryland Nursing School during the winter of 1928, returning to Annapolis in July to finish up in the Annapolis Emergency Hospital nursing school, reorganized under Superintendent Elizabeth A. Gallery. A few

Annapolis nurses, however, transferred to other nursing schools after the fire or dropped their vocation. Two senior nurses who completed their training in Baltimore came back to Annapolis for the traditional graduation ceremonies in May.

With the promise of a doubled patient load when the annex opened, Miss Gallery, the medical staff and the board agreed to restructure and upgrade the training school to meet state board requirements and attract new students. They also improved the nurses' living quarters by building an $8,100 annex onto the rear of the Nurses' Home, thus adding eight beds, an assembly room and classrooms. Twenty nurses felt themselves fortunate to share two large bathrooms and gave card parties to raise money for redecorating.

Preliminary reorganization of the training school curriculum added subjects such as chemistry, nursing ethics, drugs and solutions, surgical procedures, surgical and medical emergencies, management and history of nursing to the course load. Instructors continued to be drawn from the ranks of local physicians, with Dr. C.R. Winterode of Crownsville State Hospital coming in to lecture on mental diseases.

Following a three-month probationary period, student nurses were on duty from 7:30 a.m. to 7:30 or 8 p.m. They spent three to nine hours a week in class and had two hours free during the day for meals. They were given one afternoon off during the week and a half-day on Sunday, and were allowed three weeks vacation a year. For what must have seemed like almost constant duty, the students received $10 a month. They bought their own books and uniforms. They were housed and fed by the hospital and they received free laundry services, which must have been a particular boon because nurses' uniforms of the day were white cotton dresses, always starched, always spotless.

During its early years, the nurses' training school admitted girls as young as 17 and many with only a grade school education. After 1928, applicants were required to be between 18 and 35 years old and to have satisfactorily completed high school. Letters from a clergyman and physician attesting to their "good moral character" and "sound health" were expected. No mention was made in the school's entrance requirements, either in the 1928 annual report or the newspapers, of the fact that nurses could not be married. Presumably this was so well known a requirement as to be beyond comment. When reasons for dropping out of the training program or hospital employment were given, however, marriage appeared regularly. (The University of Maryland Nursing School did not admit or continue married students until the 1950s.) The anonymous Annapolis nursing student who had surgery for an incomplete abortion was dismissed.

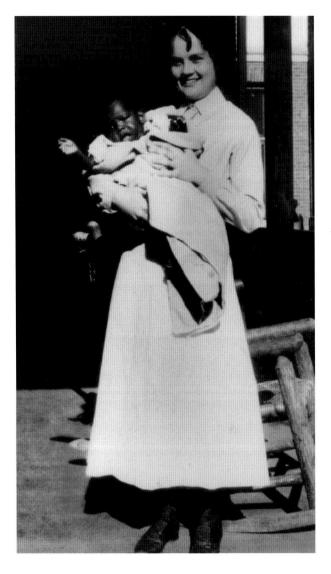

Nurse-probationer
Mary Gray with a baby
who had osteomyelitis,
1927.

When the state board again required upgrading of the training school in 1931, the hospital revised its staffing to include a superintendent, instructors, night superintendent, two teaching supervisors, operating room supervisor, anesthetist, technician and dietitian. By 1932, there were 24 student nurses, only eight of whom were local women. Most local applicants were rejected on the basis of age or poor grades. To fill the classes, a group of students was accepted from a North Carolina hospital forced to close by the Depression.

As the state's curriculum for nurses' training became more and more definitive through the early 1930s, Annapolis students, limited in their exposure to the cases of a comparatively small community hospital, found it difficult to obtain the breadth of experience required. They went regularly to Baltimore for classes and duty in specialties not often seen at the Annapolis Emergency Hospital. By 1933, qualified local women were more apt to enroll in a large municipal hospital nursing school for their entire training than stay near home and suffer the inconvenience of moving back and forth from town to city.

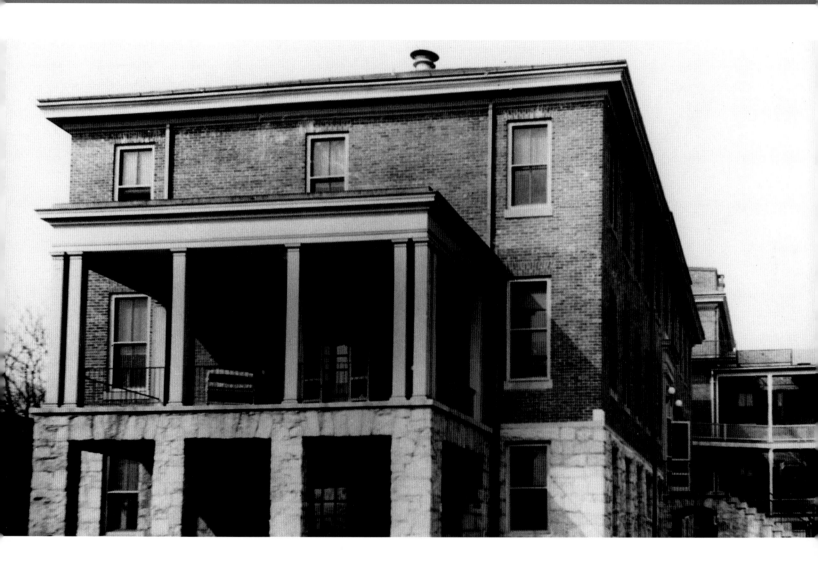

Throughout the 1920s, nurses had been in short supply, but early in the Depression the career seemed more attractive to young women and the profession became overcrowded just as hospitals were cutting back on staff or even closing. By 1933, the state board cut back the number of students allowed in small hospital training schools. The Annapolis Emergency Hospital had only eight students that year and Chief of Staff Walton H. Hopkins suggested that the hospital would be better off closing the school and hiring graduate nurses. The school closed in 1935.

The completely equipped and furnished annex opened on November 14, 1930, increasing the hospital's capacity to 100 patients. The dispensary, by 1931 being called the "accident room," the women's ward and a new children's ward were decorated and furnished by members of the community, including Dr. J. Willis Martin, chief of staff in 1931, the Zonta Club and the Children's Hospital Club.

In 1931, Dr. Martin initiated the procedure of having staff doctors rotate monthly duty in

The new 1928 annex and the porches on the back of the main building before landscaping by the Four Rivers Garden Club, c.1928.

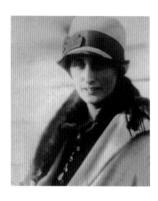

Dr. Emily H. Wilson c.1925. For many years, Dr. Wilson was the only physician in south county.

the accident room, which was, he said, "fully equipped to care for any and all kinds of emergency work" with "medical attention that is equal to any obtainable elsewhere." The X-ray department, staffed part-time by Dr. Eugene Flippen of the University of Maryland Hospital, and with a full-time technician, Miss Jane Derbyshire, processed 1,406 examinations in 1931 and received high marks for quality. Miss Derbyshire's duties also included the laboratory, under the direction of Dr. Hugh Spencer, University of Maryland pathologist. Upon the scheduled inspection by the American College of Surgeons, Dr. Martin felt confident that the Annapolis Emergency Hospital would be accredited. In 1934, the American College of Surgeons gave the institution full approval for complying with its rigorous standards. Although granted for only one year, the long-sought certificate was a source of great pride in the hospital community. In 1937, the hospital received "Grade A" approval from the American College of Surgeons.

By 1931, the hospital was feeling the effects of the Depression. While the patient load for October 1930 to October 1931 had dropped more than 8 percent compared with the year ending October 1929, just after the stock market crash, the number of free patients increased by 9 percent and the average hospital stay jumped from eight to 13 days. The death rate for admitted patients increased from the 1928–1929 figure of 2.7 percent to 4.3 percent. Births decreased slightly from 156 in 1929 to 148 in 1931. It appears from these statistics that the people of Anne Arundel County may have been less inclined to seek hospital care and may have been sicker when they did so.

The fall of 1931 also showed a marked increase in infectious diseases. Typhoid fever,

traced to a human carrier in the county (a "Typhoid Mary") and scarlet fever among children in Eastport, West Annapolis and Millersville caused concern. It was hospital policy not to admit contagious diseases such as tuberculosis, but infectious disease cases were admitted and many of the critically ill typhoid patients were hospitalized. The need for an isolation ward to care for patients with contagious diseases in the hospital was brought up again in 1932, the second year in which the patient death rate stood at 4.3 percent of admissions.

The Depression's effect on Anne Arundel County residents was less severe than that experienced by workers in Baltimore City or industrial western Maryland, but the nutrition and health care of many families in the hospital's service area declined significantly during the period. Most people in Anne Arundel County lived in rural areas, with truck farming and the seafood industry their primary occupations. Residents of Annapolis were cushioned by the various forms of government, especially the Naval Academy, which, with reasonably stable salaries, supported not only their own employees but those employed by local businesses. This is not to say that the county escaped the hard times of the 1930s, but for many, the causes of their troubles were only exacerbated by the national crisis. Decreased demand for truck produce and a general decline in the Bay's seafood industry were long-range problems.

The Annapolis Emergency Hospital inpatient population increased from 1,269 in 1930 to almost 2,000 in 1940. A marked rise in free service occurred in 1934 when over 71 percent of that year's patients could not pay for their care. In the second half of the decade, the number of free patients

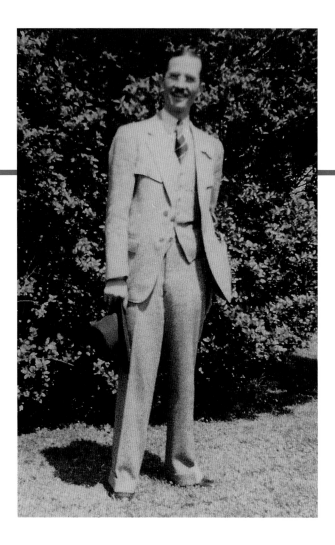

dropped to about one-third of the annual total. The Board of State Aid and Charities covered much of the cost of free patients. The average stay also dropped slightly to seven days per patient in 1940, and the hospital's expenses leveled off at the end of the decade to just under $76,000 a year. It appeared, by the start of the new decade, that service and cost were reasonably contained. No one reckoned on the changes that were to come.

By the late 1930s, almost all of the original physicians of the Annapolis Emergency Hospital were dead. Dr. Frank H. Thompson, who died in July 1937, was probably the last survivor of the 1902 medical staff. Over the intervening 35 years, most of that first group of community doctors had been elected chief of staff at least once; some, like Dr. George Wells (1843–1918) and Dr. James J. Murphy, had held the position for years. Several of them were Annapolis natives and graduates of the University of Maryland Medical School: Drs. Washington Clement Claude (1858–1924), Henry Roland Walton (1828–1912) and William S. Welch (1853–1935), whose son, Dr. Robert S. G. Welch, was elected chief of staff in 1938. The two Drs. Ridout, W. G. and John, had died in 1914 and 1936; and Dr. Sewell S. Hepburn had died in his car coming home from a patient visit at the age of 47 in 1921. They had guided the hospital through its early years, taught classes at the nursing school and helped their patients make the transition from home care to hospital care as medical science, and the hospital itself, grew and improved.

The new generation of physicians, which by 1937 included two women, Dr. Frances Weitzman and Dr. Emily Wilson, brought with them the technological training of 20th-century medical schools. Yet the tradition of the family practitioner remained very much alive.

"There were six generations of some families that I took care of. I knew all of their relatives and so much more about them. . . . When I went on my rounds, I took a lot of love and sympathy; there wasn't much medicine. I had a flashlight and a stethoscope. There were no antibiotics, but there was a lot of pneumonia and other infectious diseases. I [was] one of the first to rent oxygen tents and put the patients under the tents. Of course, most of the houses didn't have electricity and you couldn't have a lamp in the room because of the oxygen, so you'd have to have a flashlight to look at the patient to see whether he was turning blue or not!"

Dr. Emily Wilson, September 18, 1991

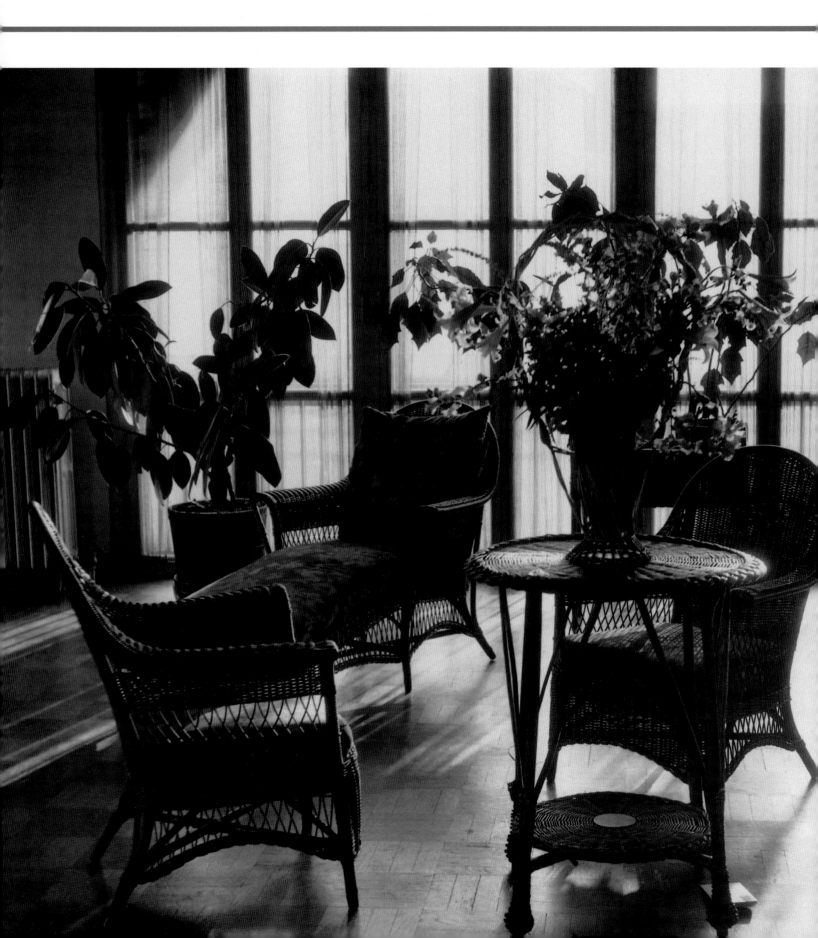

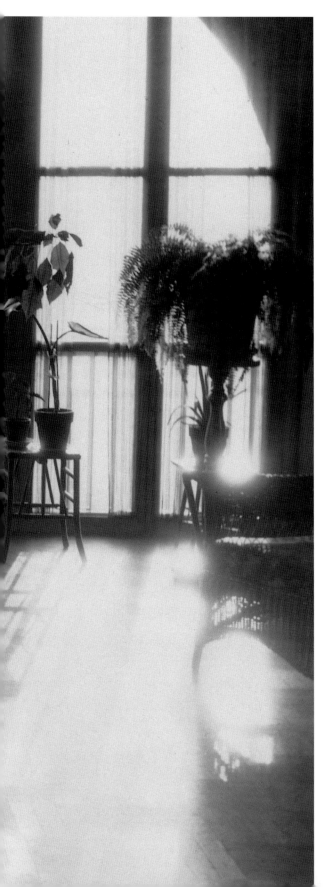

The European war that broke out in 1939 was a harbinger of the upheaval to come. For the Annapolis area, the immediate effect was jobs: increased employment at the Naval Academy and, in Eastport, the building of PT boats for Great Britain and the Soviet Union under President Franklin D. Roosevelt's Lend-Lease Program.

The pages of the *Evening Capital* during 1940 and early 1941 reflect the country's anxiety over the war and preparations for active participation. Fort Meade was resurrected as an army training and staging facility, recruiting officers from the Navy accepted enlistments of local boys, and the Annapolis Emergency Hospital was designated a training center for Red Cross nurses' aides.

The hospital admitted 2,359 patients between October 1940 and September 1941 and treated 2,842 cases in its outpatient department, or accident room. That year, 366 babies were born in the hospital. The nursing shortage continued to be a serious problem; nurses' duty hours were increased, and practical nurses and aides were hired in greater numbers. At one point during 1941, the Board of Managers even considered closing part of the hospital but compromised by curtailing the number of patients. The medical staff recommended a number of equipment purchases, including a new $10,000 X-ray machine, and the board considered, very briefly, building another addition onto the hospital. The managers finally did agree to the purchase of new operating room equipment and furnishings for wards and private rooms, but deferred the question of new construction because of the "rising costs of materials and priority difficulties." This was not the time, they felt, to be committed to an expansion program.

The renovated sun parlor on the second floor of the main building, 1928.

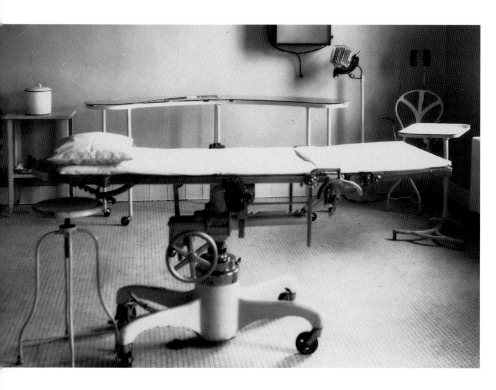

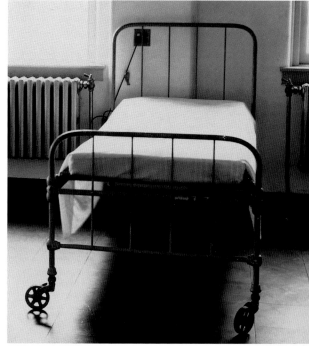

The modern operating room, c.1928.

This iron bed in the new annex had wheels but no crank to raise the head or foot, c.1928.

Nursery, c.1928, with soft mattresses and pillows!

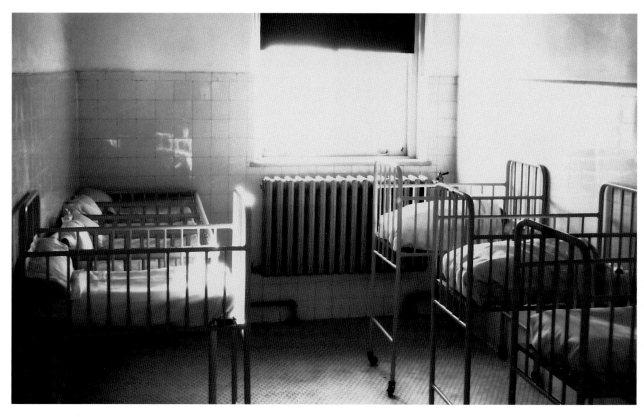

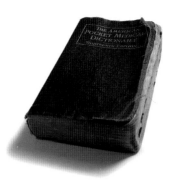

MEDICAL DICTIONARY
Courtesy of AAMC

There also was the question of who owned the hospital. William H. Labrot, a member of the advisory board and son of Sylvester Labrot, raised the question of hospital ownership at the 1941 Annapolis Emergency Hospital Association annual meeting. The hospital building and equipment were valued at more than $300,000, but the state still held title to the original land purchase and carried insurance on the physical plant. Without clear title, Mr. Labrot pointed out, the association could not borrow to enlarge the facility. This issue would continue to come up over the next six years until the General Assembly authorized conveyance of the land to the Annapolis Emergency Hospital Association in 1947. The transfer took place on February 3, 1948.

A special meeting of the Annapolis Emergency Hospital Association was called in January 1942 to authorize the appointment of three persons—one each from the Board of Managers, the medical staff and the advisory board—to work with the county health officer, William J. French and Col. John deP. Douw, county civil defense officer, as a defense emergency committee. Colonel Douw, former mayor of Annapolis and county commissioner and, for many years a member of the hospital advisory board, died in August 1942.

Another longtime hospital worker, Mrs. Margaret V. Basil, resigned in 1942. She had served as treasurer of the hospital from 1931 and had been the hospital's business manager for much of that time, carefully watching over the books through the Depression years.

Honored guests at the dinner celebrating the 40th anniversary of the hospital in 1942 were Anna Cresap and Emma Feldmeyer, the two surviving founders. During the annual meeting that followed, they heard Miss Mabel Merrick, the superintendent, give the year's statistics: 2,741 patients admitted, of whom well over one-third were children; 1,220 operations performed; 510 babies born; average length of stay, seven days. It must have given these women tremendous satisfaction to see realized the vision they had so long ago.

Amendments to the association bylaws passed in 1942 prohibited individuals or their families, on the medical staff or employed at the hospital, from serving on the Board of Managers and limited board members to two three-year terms, with reelection possible after a one-year hiatus.

The limitation of service meant the end of the "Lady Board" as it had existed from the beginning of the association. Over the years, the reelection of members whose terms had expired had become almost routine, with new women elected only at the death or resignation of a previous member. One of the first casualties of the new amendment was Selda V. Miller, a board member for almost 20 years and president for 14 years, who retired in 1943.

Just over 68,000 people lived in Anne Arundel County in 1940, about 80 percent of them in rural surroundings and almost half of them under the age of 25. But by 1943, these figures had begun to change, and change dramatically. The northern part of the county and the area around Fort Meade felt the impact of families drawn to Baltimore war industries and the military buildup. In Annapolis, the Post Graduate School of the Naval Academy brought in officers and their families, many of whom winterized the summer homes in vacation communities along the shore and moved in for the dura-

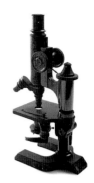

EARLY MICROSCOPE
Courtesy of Dr. Gerard Church

tion. Some of their medical needs would be met by the Naval Hospital at the academy, but many of them, along with civilian personnel in the war effort, would turn to the Annapolis Emergency Hospital for care.

For the hospital, on the other hand, the war meant severe staffing problems. Young nurses headed overseas as soon as they graduated from school. Like community hospitals across the country, the Annapolis Emergency Hospital hired nurses' aides, trained in basic procedures, to supplement the registered nurses whenever possible. Navy wives with nursing training and married alumnae of the hospital's training school were welcomed as the shortage worsened. Patients who could afford the cost often hired private-duty nurses to attend them in the hospital as well as at home. The advantages of private-duty work in both salary and working conditions continued to draw many nurses away from regular hospital employment.

Fortunately, the community continued its unfailing support. Mrs. Annie Stallings repaired and recycled hospital linens, as she

had for more than 25 years, and the ladies of the area still brought in their jams and preserves, pickles and fresh eggs to perk up the hospital diet. Church and civic groups contributed money for special equipment; the Naval Academy Women's Club, for example, donated $300 for an isolation cubicle in the children's ward. During the summer of 1944, high school girls were trained as dietitian's aides and assisted with the preparation of salads, desserts and special diets.

In 1943, the hospital admitted 2,577 patients, a 10 percent increase over the previous year and a terrific strain on the staff. The dispensary treated 2,233 cases. The hospital's costs in 1943 totaled more than $139,000, almost $13,000 more than its income. At a time when perhaps 80 percent of the residents of Maryland's counties made less than $2,000 a year, these figures were impressive.

In August 1944, the Board of Managers recognized the hospital's growth by hiring an administrator to manage the physical plant, finances and general operation. The first administrator was Loran S. Messick, formerly

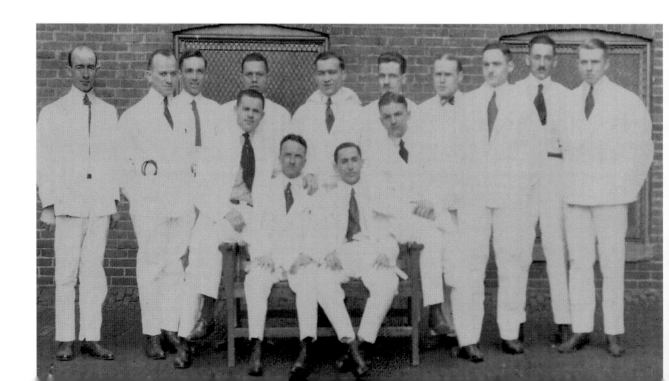

Dr. J. Willis Martin (second from right), chief of the medical staff in 1931, joins other members of the medical staff, c.1930.

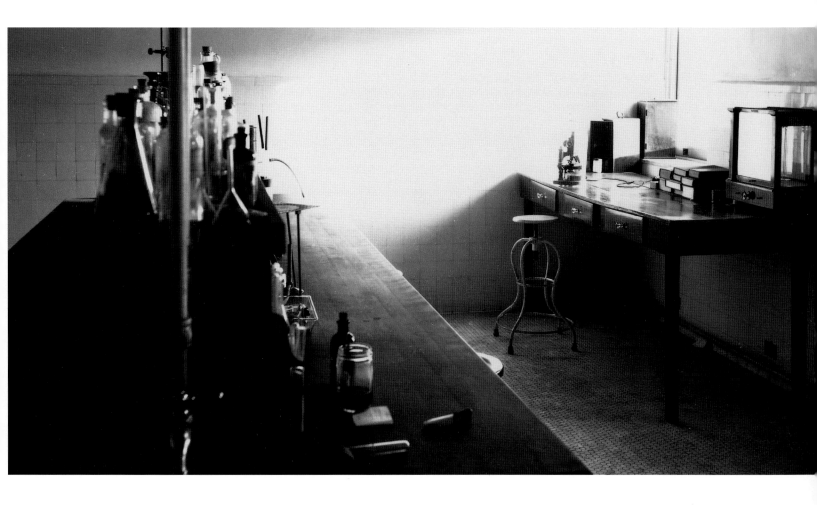

assistant superintendent of Salisbury's Peninsula General Hospital. He set to work immediately with a major housecleaning and refurbishing.

Also during 1944, the hospital chief of staff, Dr. Walton Hopkins, secured the round-the-clock services of interns from the Naval Hospital to assist the medical staff, principally in the dispensary, which again treated roughly 2,000 cases. There were, in 1944, 14 physicians (three of them women) on the active staff of the hospital, with three physicians from the academy as courtesy staff with limited privileges and 12 specialists from Baltimore as consultants. The regular nursing

staff was composed of 23 full- and part-time registered nurses. The support and technical staff included a bookkeeper, record librarian, two admitting officers, two X-ray and laboratory technicians, a dietitian, a nurse-anesthetist, three practical nurses and four paid nurses' aides.

Maternity patients' costs were $7 per day for a private room, $5.50 for a semi-private room and $4.50 a day for ward patients, with a $10 delivery room charge and $1 per day nursery charge for each infant. Medical and surgical patients paid $7 and $8 a day for private rooms, $5.50 for semi-private rooms and $3.50 for ward beds. Patients unable to pay

Laboratory, c.1928.

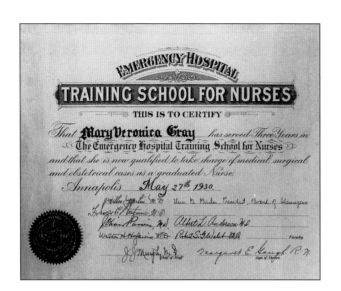

were housed free in the ward beds. All patients paid additional fees for medicines, X-rays, special tests and treatments, and anesthesia. There were no semi-private rooms for male patients.

Hospital admissions in 1944 totaled 2,025, over half of them surgical patients. There were 406 obstetrical patients. The average daily patient population was 50 and the average stay was eight days. There were 317 live births recorded, almost 11,000 laboratory examinations and 912 operations. The hospital's new fluoroscopy machine was used for 92 examinations.

Enlarged Nurses' Home, 1930s.

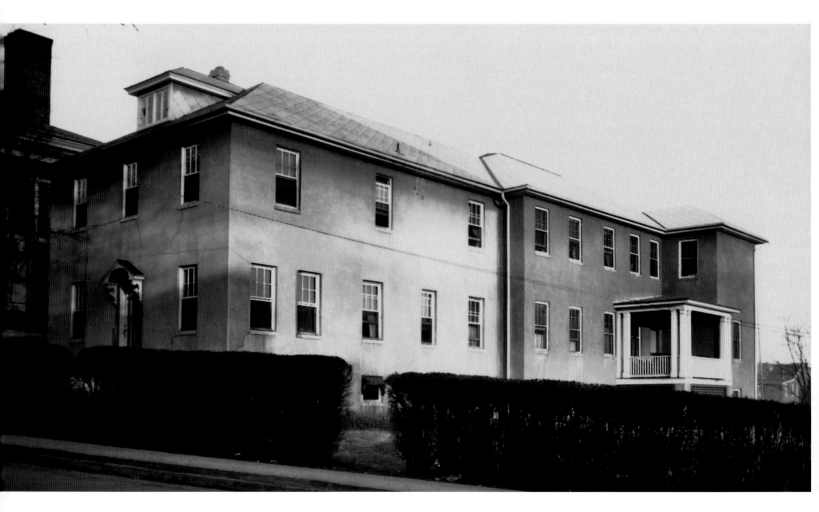

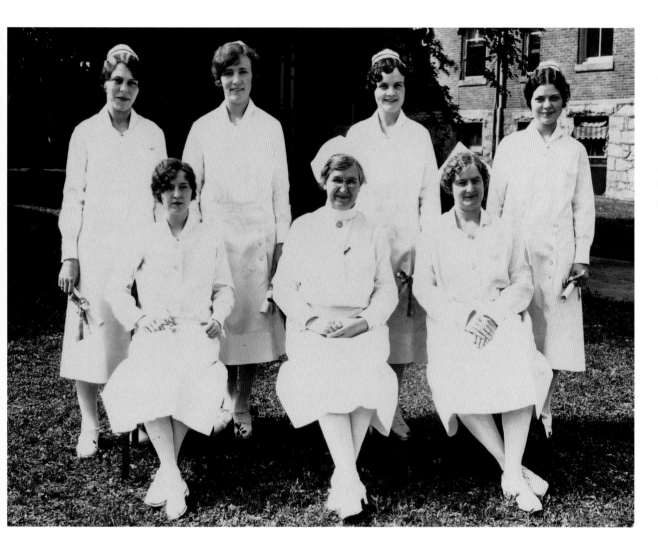

Annapolis Emergency Hospital Training School for Nurses graduating class of 1930. Seated (left to right): Ellen Evans; Miss Elizabeth Gallery, superintendent; Miss Marguerite Gough, director of the nursing school. Standing (left to right): Minna Sattmary, Katherine Tyler, Mary Gray, Marian Richardson.

In October 1944, the Women's Auxiliary of the Annapolis Emergency Hospital formed under the leadership of President Selda V. Miller, former president of the Board of Managers. The stated objective of the organization was "to give more people in the community an opportunity to take an active part in the hospital." Several former board members were involved, including Miss Nyce Feldmeyer and Mrs. Walter B. Tardy. The Auxiliary appointed committees of ways and means, membership and house furnishings and set about raising the money and providing the services that have made it, over the succeeding years, such an important part of the hospital family.

A proposal in 1944 to change the name of the institution to the Annapolis General Hospital was made and set aside for the moment. The original critical care concept had long been outdated; the Annapolis Emergency Hospital was, in fact, a general hospital offering a wide range of care and services. But the name change would have to wait for another time—and other changes.

When I came to the hospital in 1949, it was a small place, just 60 beds or so, and there were still open wards.

When I first got here, I went to see all the physicians in town. Don Hooker and George Basil welcomed me. George said that the older physicians had opposed him, but he came anyway and made a go of it and I could be a success, too!

The staff wasn't very sophisticated, so John Rich got physicians from Johns Hopkins and the University of Maryland to be chiefs of service. A couple of us 'Young Turks' thought we'd convince the 'Old Guard' that we had something to say, and I became the first local chief of medicine in 1952. I resigned in 1961.

During that time, we brought a number of new doctors into the hospital. Bill Thomas was the first full-time radiology doctor; before he came we had a man come down from Baltimore twice a week to read X-rays. Wally Alden was the first chief of pathology. Before he came, I had one case where I badly wanted an autopsy, so I had to drive up to Crownsville to pick up a pathologist there and bring him back here to do the autopsy.

We also got one of our first trained surgeons other than Don Hooker—Jess Wilkins. Before then, the general practitioners did their own surgeries. A number of medical subspecialists came to town, too—cardiologists Gerry Church and Bob Bierne, anesthesiologist Jack Lyons and oncologist Stan Watkins, to name a few.

We knew all the nurses well; we knew their competency levels. We trained some of our nurses to do resuscitations and administer medicine. We were one of the first coronary care units in the nation that operated without house staff. It was a real friendly, personal atmosphere.

Perspective...

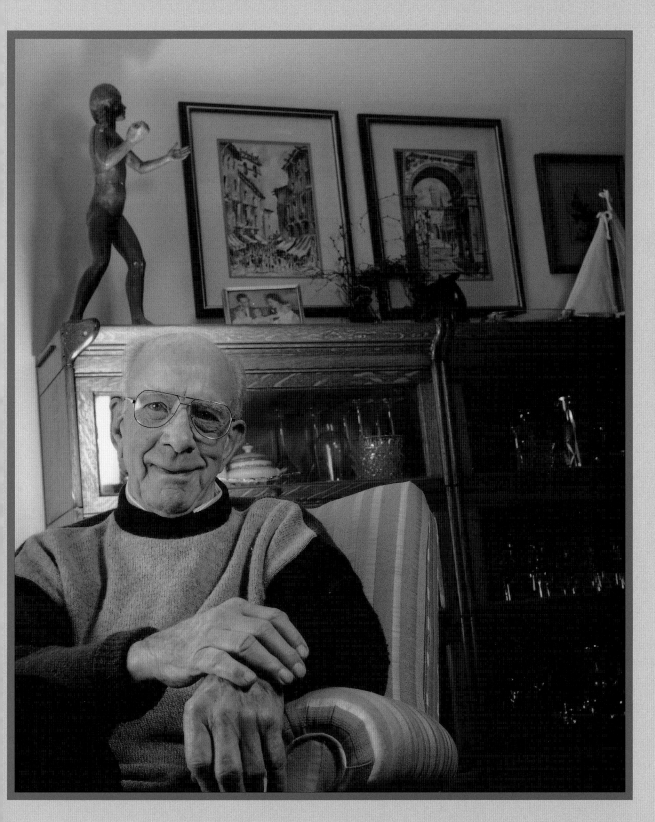

Dr. Frank M. Shipley

Established internal medicine practice in Annapolis, 1949

Medical staff president, 1956-1958

I attended Ohio State University and later Howard University, where I received an R.N. degree from its Freedman's Hospital Nursing School and then completed my medical training.

I had a love of medicine, and I wanted to help people. I met my husband [Aris T. Allen, M.D.] at Howard; when he graduated from medical school he started a family medicine practice in Annapolis in 1945. After I graduated, I joined him here. We had two sons by that time. The two of us thought we could conquer the world!

We had our medical office in Annapolis near the Church Circle post office, and we saw our patients there or went to their homes. We couldn't join the medical staff until the mid-1950s, because the medical society wouldn't accept blacks at that time. So we delivered babies at home or at Dr. Johnson's private hospital on Northwest Street. We'd have to refer our sick patients to Freedman's Hospital (part of Howard University) or send them up to Johns Hopkins. We referred our surgical patients to local surgeons. One time, the surgeon asked Aris to scrub in and stand in the OR while he was operating on one of our patients. We received hate letters for that!

It was a really difficult time. As a woman, it was tough, but it was doubly hard as a black woman. When I first joined the medical staff, I obeyed every rule. You had to prove yourself; you had to be better. The first time I was on call at the hospital emergency room, I sat home all day waiting, but I didn't get any calls. Dr. Shipley found out that the nurse on duty was calling him instead when white patients came in! He really gave them hell for that!

But things smoothed out after awhile, and it quieted down. Annapolis was a good place to practice medicine and a good place to live. I can't imagine any other career. I truly love Anne Arundel Medical Center and feel very proud to have been a member of the medical staff.

Perspective...

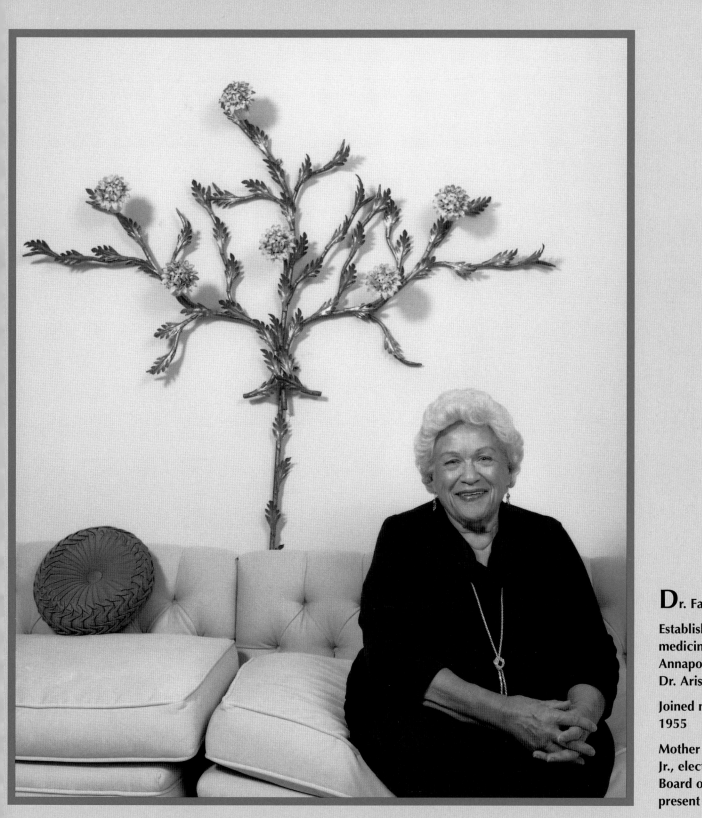

Dr. Faye Watson Allen

Established family medicine practice in Annapolis with husband Dr. Aris T. Allen, 1950

Joined medical staff, 1955

Mother of Aris T. Allen, Jr., elected to AAHS Board of Trustees, 2000-present

The end of World War II initiated a period of population growth in Anne Arundel County unparalleled since its founding in 1649. A placid, agricultural backwater of just over 68,000 residents in 1940, by 1950 Anne Arundel had a population of more than 117,000 in its 416 square miles. The districts south of Baltimore City changed, almost overnight it seemed, to bustling suburbs. The county would never again have the rural peacefulness of its preceding 300 years.

Many of the industrial workers and military families, drawn to the county by the war effort, stayed. Servicemen returning after the war found that new roads (Ritchie Highway had opened in 1940) and the affordable housing of the postwar Federal Housing Administration and Veterans Administration programs made it possible for them to work in the city and rear their families in the older waterfront communities along the Severn and Magothy rivers or in new developments of single family homes. Harundale opened in 1950, followed by Hillsmere, Chartwell, Maryland City and more than 30 smaller subdivisions in the Glen Burnie area. By 1960, the county would be home to more than 206,000 people, three times its 1940 population.

The rush to the suburbs created jobs in construction, merchandising, services and, eventually, in new industries. Before 1948, only 12 businesses in the county employed more than 100 workers; the Naval Academy, with 2,000 employees, was the largest. The opening of the National Plastics Corporation plant in Odenton in 1948, followed in 1951 by a Westinghouse facility near the new Friendship Airport (now BWI), provided employment to local workers and encouraged others to move to the area.

Medical advances of the war era, most

notably the use of antibiotics, underlined the general public belief in the efficacy of modern medicine and its practice within a hospital setting. The Board of Managers, the advisory board and physicians of the Annapolis Emergency Hospital may not have comprehended the full extent of the changes that would come after the war, but they certainly anticipated that greater demands would be put on their hospital. In 1945, they began planning for renovations and an enlargement of the building on Franklin Street. The news in September 1945 that the army would soon demobilize 25,000 nurses brought hope that the hospital finally could obtain an adequate nursing staff.

The annual meeting of the Annapolis Emergency Hospital Association in November 1945 introduced a major change in the hospital's management. Three men were elected to fill the place of outgoing board members. For the first time since Mayor Charles DuBois's brief stint as president of the board in 1902, the Board of Managers of the hospital included both men and women. The first male board members were T. Carroll Worthington, an Annapolis realtor and appraiser, John Baldwin Rich, an investment banker, and Rev. Robert L. Jones, rector of St. Anne's. Mr. Rich was promptly elected president of the board and just as promptly set about making the operation of the hospital efficient, controlled and thoroughly professional. There were some who felt his management was abrupt and even occasionally dictatorial, but few would challenge his effect on the hospital's well-being and almost all would praise him for his success and his many years of hard work for the hospital.

A concentrated campaign to increase contributions and paid memberships in the association to cover yearly deficits in the hospital's

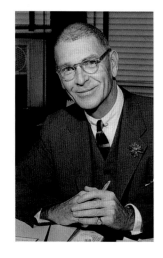

John B. Rich, 1959.

"I'd say he spent 60 percent of his time looking after things. There wasn't anything that happened over in that hospital in those days that Jack Rich didn't know about."

William J. McWilliams
January 15, 1992
Past President
Board of Managers

A Change in Direction
1945 - 1958

budget netted more than $32,000 by November 1946. The Annapolis metropolitan area donated almost half of that amount, but residents of the other county districts, civic groups, the Severn River Naval Command and the hospital's own family of physicians, nurses and workers all made substantial contributions to putting the hospital on sound financial footing. Only then, said Albert H. MacCarthy, chairman of the campaign, could the hospital solicit "memorial donations for the expansion and improvement of facilities of the hospital and the creation of an endowment fund."

The 1946 annual meeting again considered a more appropriate name for the hospital. This time "Anne Arundel County Hospital" was discussed and put aside. The association did vote to amend its constitution to reflect the altered mission of the hospital and the word "emergency" was struck. The stated purpose

Busy medical ward, c.1950s.

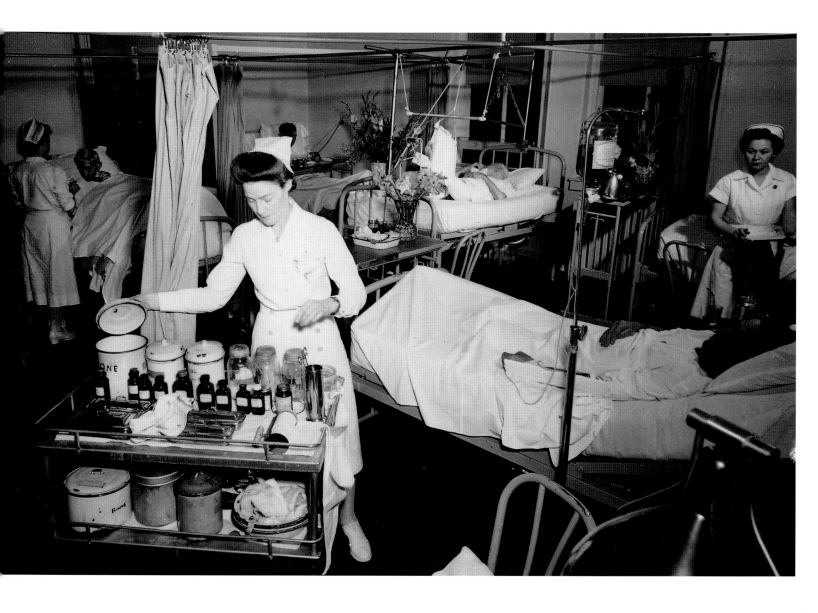

of the corporation was now to "establish and conduct a general hospital at Annapolis, Maryland." The association also amended the constitution to provide for the organization of the medical staff under bylaws that would spell out the qualifications for admitting new physicians to the staff. Appointments of staff physicians would continue to be the province of the board, upon the recommendation of the medical staff. Because there was no actual provision in the Annapolis Emergency Hospital Association constitution for the election of an advisory board, as had been customary under the lady board, Mr. Rich announced that henceforth the advisers would be appointed by the Board of Managers.

Admissions of 2,705 patients during 1946 seemed to justify the board's anxiety to get business in order and plan for enlargement. Doctors performed 1,084 operations, 438 of them designated as major, and treated more than 2,100 patients in the accident room. Dr. Frank E. Champo came to Annapolis Emergency Hospital from Peninsula General in Salisbury in December 1945 as the first resident physician in the emergency room.

Loran S. Messick resigned as administrator in October 1946. The need to fill his position provoked no dissension, as the administrator's role grew with the hospital. Increasingly complex finances and relationships with government agencies and private insurers, as well as the general management of the hospital's 100 or so employees, warranted full-time attention. No longer could these duties be handled by committees of the volunteer board or by the superintendent of nurses.

Sherrill S. Adams, who accepted the position of administrator in January 1947, was an Annapolis resident retired from the Navy Medical Service Corps. Prior to coming to Annapolis Emergency Hospital, he had been for two years the property and accounting officer of the Naval Academy Hospital.

Mr. Adams encouraged the new hospital Auxiliary in its first efforts to provide patients with a more pleasant hospital stay. The book cart, from which patients could borrow reading material, and the flower service, which tended to patients' gift bouquets and plants, brought friendly members of the community into hospital rooms. Their smiles and bedside chats were usually a welcome diversion in patients' daily routines.

Patient services increased across the board in 1947. Most notable was the 39 percent increase in births over the 1946 figure. Lab and X-ray exams now numbered in the thousands per year and accident room visits were up almost 25 percent. The total number of patients treated during the hospital's accounting year ending September 30, 1947, passed the 5,000 mark and was climbing steadily. Although the cost of providing these services had doubled since 1944, revenues kept pace and the hospital showed a net profit of almost $8,000, which Treasurer Albert H. MacCarthy credited to more efficient management and the greater volume of business.

Dr. Harold Bohlman, consulting orthopedist, opened an orthopedic clinic at Annapolis Emergency Hospital in 1947, and a cancer clinic, sponsored by the Maryland branch of the American Cancer Society and the county health department, met at regular intervals.

Improvements to the interior of the building and refurbishing of the delivery room and private rooms during 1948 were funded largely by private individuals and local civic organizations, including Mr. and Mrs. W. H. Labrot, Kneseth Israel Congregation, Annapolis Jewish Charities, the Annapolis branch of the National Council of Jewish Women, B'nai B'rith, the Jewish War Veterans and the Annapolis Lions Club. The Annapolis Lodge of Elks provided an oxygen tent, resuscitator and electrocardiograph, and the Annapolis and Anne Arundel County chapter, National Foundation for Infantile Paralysis, gave a chest-type respirator. Two private rooms were added and plans were made to enclose the porches for additional rooms.

The hospital's occupancy rate that year rose to 74 percent. More than 5,800 people were treated, with admissions outnumbering accident room cases for the first time. There were 552 births and 114 deaths. As many as 92 patients were lodged in the hospital at one time that year and beds in the halls were becoming common. While most patients came to the hospital from the Annapolis and Eastport areas, south county, the northern and southern shores of the Severn River, and the Odenton-Gambrills area, there were patients from Washington and Baltimore (presumably visitors to Anne Arundel County), Prince George's, Calvert and Howard counties, Harundale, Linthicum, Pasadena and a few from the Eastern Shore. This was, of course, before the Chesapeake Bay Bridge was built, and Eastern Shore residents needing care beyond that offered by their local hospitals were generally taken directly to teaching hospitals in Baltimore.

In 1948, Anne Arundel County's appropriation to cover indigent and accident patients amounted to $5,000 per year, the city's, $1,000. The county also set aside $12,000 for the hospital to draw from during periods in which there was a deficit between the expenses of caring for state-aid patients and

Black men's ward, early 1940s.

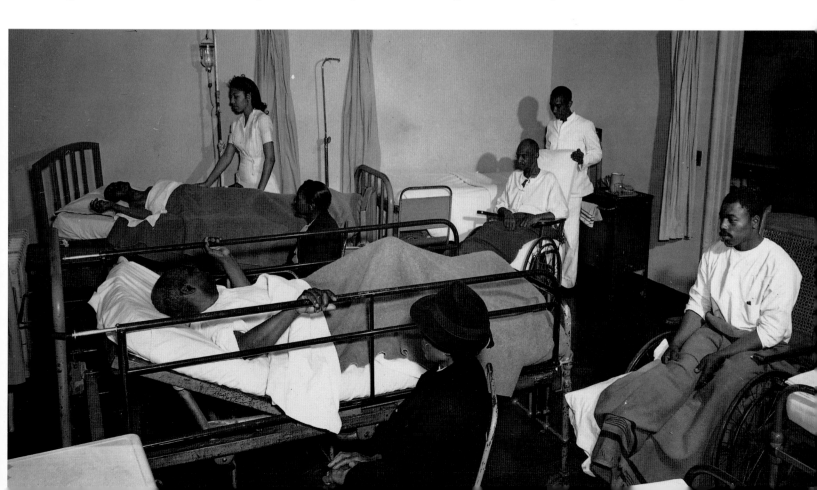

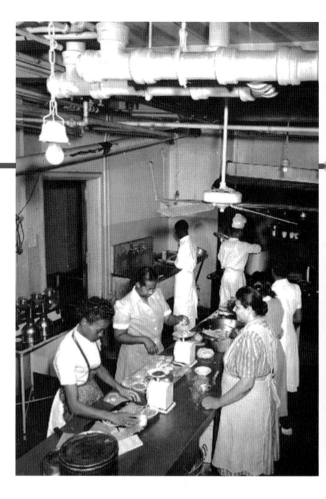

Kitchen in the basement of the 1928 annex, c.1943.

the receipt of state money. For many years, the state had paid a standard *per diem* rate for the care of those patients who were certified as in need of public support.

A major reorganization of the medical staff during 1948, under the new bylaws adopted in 1947, divided the staff into four services: gynecology, surgery, obstetrics and medicine. The respective chiefs of these services were Baltimore physicians Dr. John D. Dumler, Dr. Robert C. Kimberly, Dr. John Whitridge, Jr. and Dr. Harry F. Klinefelter.

Local physicians were admitted to practice in the hospital under one or more of these services depending upon their qualifications and experience. Dr. Robert S. G. Welch remained as chief of staff. By 1949, the regular staff numbered 16, with six courtesy staff members and 26 physicians from Baltimore and Washington on the consulting staff.

By 1949, the 11-member Board of Managers was comprised of six men and five women. Cognizant of both projected county population figures and the hospital's present high occupancy rate, they initiated a major fundraising campaign to finance the imperative expansion of the hospital's facilities.

A fundraising and public relations firm, Charles A. Haney and Associates, Inc. of Newtonville, Massachusetts, had been hired in 1948 to assess the amount and kind of enlargement necessary and present a plan for fundraising. The Haney report, dated April 17, 1949, recommended a number of changes, some minor, many major, including a new pharmacy, separation of medical and surgical patients, provision for black maternity patients and children, a modern operating suite, maternity department, X-ray unit, laboratory and accident room. The current hospi-

tal was not only too small, the report said, but its layout and space allotment were far below the accepted standards for a modern hospital. Haney and Associates proposed a 40–50 bed addition, with both private and semi-private rooms, and an almost total reorganization of the existing facility.

With these facts and recommendations, the hospital's management took its case to the people of Anne Arundel County with a lavish brochure and a plea for financing. The community was encouraged to designate its gifts for specific rooms or services as memorials. The total cost of the addition and renovations was estimated at $775,000.

The Summerfield Baldwin, Jr. Foundation pledged $175,000 to the building fund plus a $200,000 endowment, contingent upon the successful completion of the campaign. The income from the endowment was earmarked for maintenance and upkeep of the new wing. The Foundation also covered the cost of the campaign.

The board expected to receive one-third the

HOSPITAL GETS NEW NAME!

EVENING CAPITAL
November 22, 1949
Headline referring to changing name to
Anne Arundel General Hospital

total projected cost of the building project, or about $250,000, from the federal government under the provisions of the 1946 Hospital Survey and Construction Act, also called the Hill-Burton Bill. The community would need to contribute $350,000.

The community fundraising drive was launched on June 8, 1949. Just over five weeks later, on July 19, campaign workers crowded in front of the hospital to watch the drive's poster thermometer rise over the top with a splash of red paint. They had collected pledges of more than $500,000!

The annual meeting of the Annapolis Emergency Hospital Association in November 1949 celebrated the successful fundraising campaign and, finally, brought the hospital's official title into keeping with the reality of the institution. A bylaw adopted at that meeting formally changed the name to Anne Arundel General Hospital. "Anne Arundel" because, as President John B. Rich pointed out, the hospital's service area included the whole county, not just Annapolis, and more than two-thirds of the pledges made in the recent campaign had come from outside Annapolis; "General" because the hospital was no longer just an emergency facility but afforded a wide range of medical specialties. Underscoring the name change was another change in the bylaws adding pediatrics, orthopedics, and eye, ear, nose and throat to the appointed medical services of the hospital. Although the name of the hospital changed, the corporation remained the Annapolis Emergency Hospital Association.

The Board of Managers was increased to 16— 15 managers to be elected by the Annapolis Emergency Hospital Association and the 16th to be designated by the Summerfield Baldwin, Jr. Foundation as specified in its gift.

As soon as the expected federal aid allocation was received, said President Rich, construction contracts would be let and the new wing begun. The architect, James R. Edmunds, Jr., was working on revised plans. Because of the oversubscription by the public, the new wing could have an additional floor and be adequate to house all patients at the hospital's current occupancy rate.

Just as the hospital board and the community thought the new wing was a certainty, the Korean War caused a drastic reduction in the federal funds available for hospital construction. Instead of the $1.5 million allotment it expected, Maryland would be lucky to receive $750,000 to allocate among the 12 hospitals with construction proposals. With a revised cost of $1.1 million for its planned wing and renovations, Annapolis Emergency Hospital Association had expected the government's third to come to something over $365,000. But with only $750,000 total coming to Maryland, Anne Arundel General Hospital could not hope to get what it had anticipated.

The reduction and delay of federal funds, coupled with the fact that almost half of the community pledges had not been paid by November 1950, was a severe disappointment. At a period when admissions, accident room visits and births were up 11–12 percent, the delay in construction meant further overcrowding, more beds in hallways and a severe lack of comfort and amenities for patients.

The board decided to go ahead with construction on a limited basis and, at the end of November 1950, opened bids for the new boiler and power plant to be located on the southernmost corner of the hospital property. The two-story power plant, completed in August 1951, housed two 150-horsepower

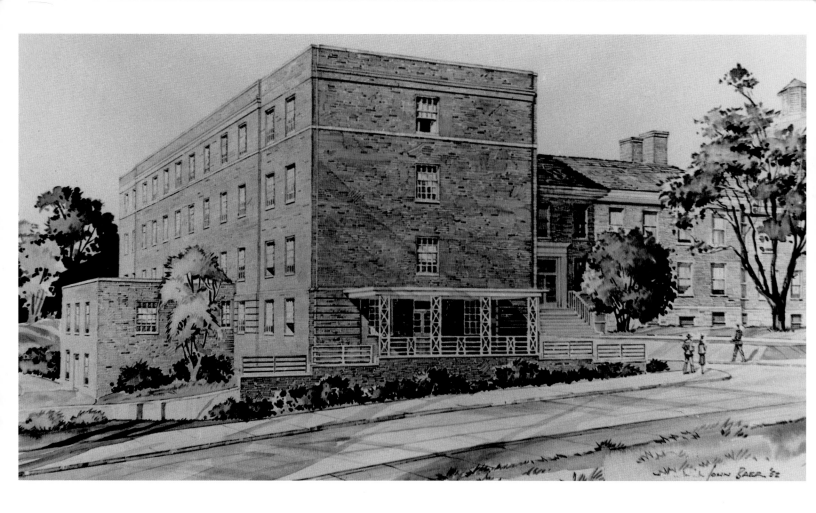

steam generators and a 60-kilowatt diesel generator for emergency electrical service. Part of the second floor became a workshop.

Also added in 1951 was a one-story, 24-bed brick annex for medical patients. Financed entirely by members of the hospital staff, the Auxiliary and friends, the $50,000 annex was named the John B. Rich Building in honor of Mr. Rich, six-year president of the Annapolis Emergency Hospital Association. At the conclusion of his two three-year terms, Mr. Rich remained on the board as the appointee of the Baldwin

Foundation and accepted the position as treasurer of the association.

With the status of the federal construction grant still unclear, the board looked for alternative funding for the expansion. In 1951, the Maryland General Assembly authorized the Anne Arundel County Commissioners to issue bonds of up to $600,000 for the hospital building fund. There was some question as to whether the state Constitution allowed this kind of bond issue, however, and the matter went into the courts for a ruling. The Court of Appeals' decision in March 1952 upheld the constitutionality of the act—the hospital could be partially financed by county bonds and the

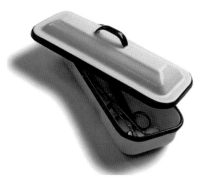

STERLIZATION TRAY C.1950
Courtesy of AAMC

county would be represented on the board by two commissioners.

Finally, on October 29, 1952, the contract for construction of the new Summerfield Baldwin, Jr. Memorial Wing was awarded to the Annapolis firm Stehle and Beans, Inc. for a bid of just over $1,143,000, the lowest bid received from the seven companies submitting them. The following Thursday, November 6, Summerfield Baldwin, Jr. climbed into a Reds Dove steam shovel and pushed the levers that dug the blade into the sod at the back of the old hospital. Construction had begun; completion was scheduled for December 31, 1953.

Governor Theodore R. McKeldin, state legislators, Anne Arundel County commissioners and Annapolis city officials joined the hospital board and friends in saluting the occasion. Dr. Emily H. Wilson, chief of the medical staff, described the improved medical services to be offered by the new wing and Rear Adm. F. C. Greaves, (M.C.) USN, inspector general of the Navy's Bureau of Medicine and Surgery, addressed the 100 or so attendees on the progress of medical science.

By 1952, the Auxiliary was becoming an important link between the hospital and the community. Its sponsorship of concerts in Annapolis by the National Symphony Orchestra or the Baltimore Symphony brought professional classical music on a regular basis to adults at evening performances and schoolchildren at special concerts during the day. During this year, the Auxiliary opened the Clothes Box, one of its most successful long-term fundraising activities, which has continued over the years to benefit both the hospital coffers and the community by recycling used clothing. Good-quality clothing and accessories have always been accept-

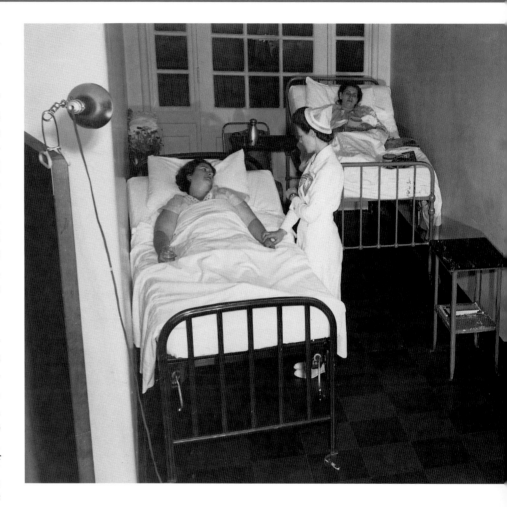

ed by the Clothes Box, with a small commission to the donor, and resold at low prices. The location of the Clothes Box has moved many times since 1952, but its patrons still seek it out.

In addition to its direct community activities, by 1952 the Auxiliary had added to its in-hospital services with radio rental for patients. Auxiliary members also transported blood between the hospital and Baltimore. Other volunteers, led by Mary M. Proskey, spent hundreds of hours sewing sheets, diapers and baby clothing for hospital use. The Auxiliary was a charter member of the Maryland Association of Hospital Auxiliaries in 1952

Nurse Ann Cole tends to patients in a hospital hallway, c.1949. Chronic overcrowding led to the construction of the John B. Rich Building.

73

The Clothes Box opened in 1952. The Auxiliary played an important role in the hospital's growth.

and by December of that year its membership had grown to 175.

By the late 1940s, young local physicians on the medical staff felt that they had the training and experience to head a service in their specialty, but it took several years to convince John Rich and the board of that. In 1948, Dr. Philip Briscoe was named the first local chief of pediatrics and four years later, Dr. Frank M. Shipley became chief of medicine, taking the post from Dr. Klinefelter of Johns Hopkins. Shortly after this, Drs. Samuel Borssuck, Stuart

Christhilf and Jess Wilkins were named as chiefs of obstetrics, gynecology and surgery. Having a chief of service whose practice was centered in Annapolis rather than in Baltimore meant daily peer review of physicians in that service and, as a result, better medicine. It also meant that the hospital would attract more well-trained young specialists. As new services were added, they were headed by local physicians.

Responding to the requests of the medical staff, Anne Arundel General Hospital began

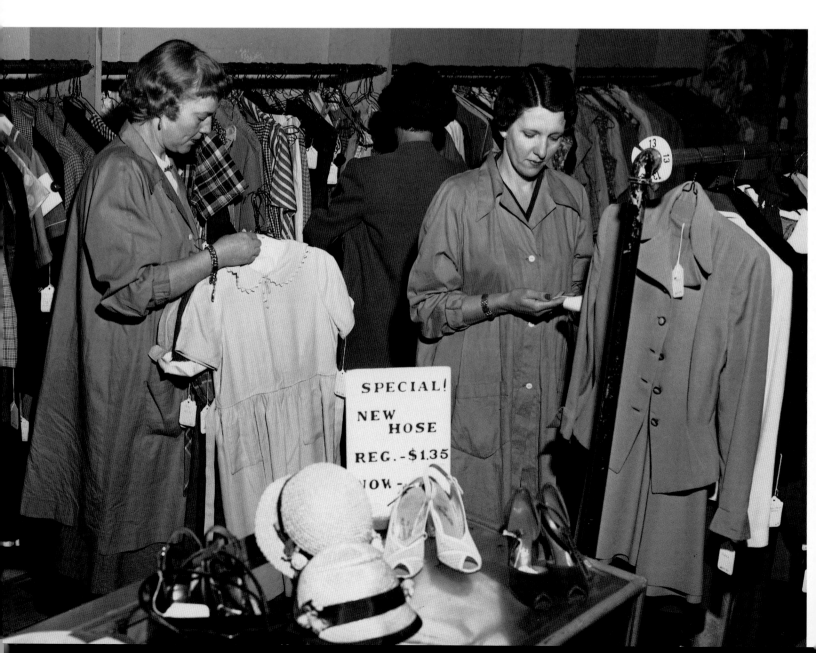

SPECIAL!
NEW HOSE
REG.-$1.35
NOW-

routine chest X-rays on admitted patients in August 1952, one of the first Maryland hospitals to do so. The Board of Managers also hired a full-time pathologist, Dr. Manning W. Alden, to run the laboratory. Lab examinations in 1952 totaled more than 38,000; by 1953, the number of exams had risen to almost 46,000 and diagnostic procedures were redefined and extended. No longer did physicians have to wait several days for the results of lab work sent to Baltimore.

Even with the new annex, hospital occupancy remained steady at 77 percent through 1952, 1953 and 1954, exceeding the recommended 75 percent maximum. Births at the hospital increased from 693 in 1952 to 777 in 1953. Population growth throughout the county continued its upward spiral. The need for the new wing became more and more intense.

In 1953, the board decided to enclose the hospital's porches for a gain of 26 beds. Construction of the Baldwin Wing progressed slowly. The Auxiliary opened a lunchtime snack bar for construction workers, which was so successful that plans were made to expand the operation in the new building.

In anticipation of the staffing needs required by the new wing, the hospital opened a school for practical nurses in June 1953. Approved by the Maryland state board, the one-year course offered lectures by the medical and nursing staffs. The 22 students admitted in 1953 ranged in age from 18 to 40; the class was racially mixed and included both men and women. Although William Weatherford graduated with the first class, by 1955 the school was composed only of women, many of whom were married. Classes were admitted each year in September and March. The first half of the year was spent learning proper care procedures and hospital routines; during the second six months, students assisted registered nurses and physicians in actual patient care.

Also in 1953, the hospital brought in a full-time physician-anesthesiologist to administer surgical and delivery anesthesia. The following year, Dr. William Thomas Belger became chief of the anesthesia service.

The new emergency instrument tray in the operating room saved its first patient in May 1954 when a Belvedere Beach woman went into cardiac arrest during a hernia operation. Dr. Elmer G. Linhardt, assisted by emergency house physician Dr. Frank E. Champo, opened her chest and massaged her heart. Within eight minutes, the patient's heart resumed a normal beat.

At this time, the operating rooms were located on the third floor of the renovated 1910 building facing Franklin Street. For many years, the rooms had no window shades in order to take full advantage of the natural light, and the children of the McWilliams family who lived across the street enjoyed hours of fascinating entertainment. They learned to recognize the various doctors and made sure everyone was at the third-floor bedroom window to catch their most interesting procedures. One of their favorite surgeons was Dr. George Basil, whose dapper dress and lighthearted jokes made him popular with hospital patients and staff as well.

After two years of routine chest X-ray screening, hospital radiologist Dr. William N. Thomas, Sr. reported at the end of 1954 that he and his associate, Dr. Robert H. Armstrong, Jr. had discovered a number of abnormalities

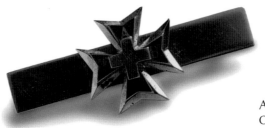

presenting no other symptoms. Twenty percent of the X-rays analyzed had shown problems such as tuberculosis, cardiovascular abnormalities and lung cancer, affording the patient the opportunity for prompt treatment and, in the case of active tuberculosis, allowing the hospital to isolate these patients immediately for the safety of other patients and hospital personnel. Dr. H. Dabney Kerr, president of the American Board of Radiology and professor emeritus of radiology of the State University of Iowa, joined the hospital as an associate in radiation therapy in 1955.

A medical library was established at the hospital in 1954 to provide the staff with access to books and periodicals of medical importance. Dedicated by the medical staff to the Annapolis Emergency Hospital Association president in tribute to the time, effort and financial assistance he had given the hospital, the library was named the Charles B. Lynch Medical Library.

Dr. Raymond L. Richardson, who joined the medical staff in December 1954, was the first African-American doctor on the staff since the death of Dr. William Bishop in 1904. Dr. Richardson was followed by Dr. Theodore H. Johnson and Drs. Aris T. and Faye Allen in 1955.

Although the hospital had treated black patients from the beginning, it did not open its delivery room to African-American mothers until 1955. Before that, black obstetricians and midwives delivered these babies at home or in office clinics or sent the mothers to Baltimore or Washington hospitals. Sometimes in an emergency, Dr. Aris Allen remembered, he would put patients in his own car and drive them to Freedman's Hospital or Johns Hopkins. Nurse Cassie Gaskins credits Mayor William U. McCready

with instituting the hospital's acceptance of black maternity patients: "Mrs. Brooks worked for Mayor McCready, and she had a daughter who was married and she was going to deliver. Well, she told Mayor McCready, 'It's a shame that my daughter has to go either to Washington or Baltimore to deliver this baby.' So he said, 'You don't have to do that, she can go to this hospital'."

Seventeen months after the laying of the cornerstone, the new Baldwin Wing opened to the public at dedication ceremonies on May 12, 1955. Summerfield Baldwin, Jr. presented the keys of the new building to Annapolis Emergency Hospital Association President Charles B. Lynch. Rev. C. Edward Berger, rector of St. Anne's Church, gave the principal address.

On May 11, the *Evening Capital* welcomed the new building with a special section devoted to the hospital, its history and personnel. County businesses placed advertisements of congratulations. All seemed to agree with President Lynch that this event was "one of the most important ever to take place in the county."

The basement of the Baldwin Wing housed a new, modern, explosion-proof operating suite with two rooms for major surgery, one for minor surgery and a postoperative recovery room. Walls, patient drapes and the doctors' and nurses' uniforms were all colored a pastel green to reduce glare and shadow-proof lights were installed to illuminate the operating tables. Two registered nurses assisted at each operation.

Also in the new basement were two delivery and two labor rooms for maternity patients. The maternity ward upstairs featured a tem-

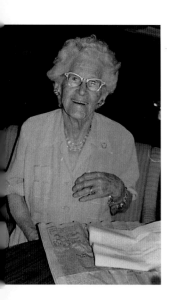

Mary M. Proskey in 1975, with papers removed from the cornerstone of the 1928 building, constructed when she was a member of the Board of Managers.

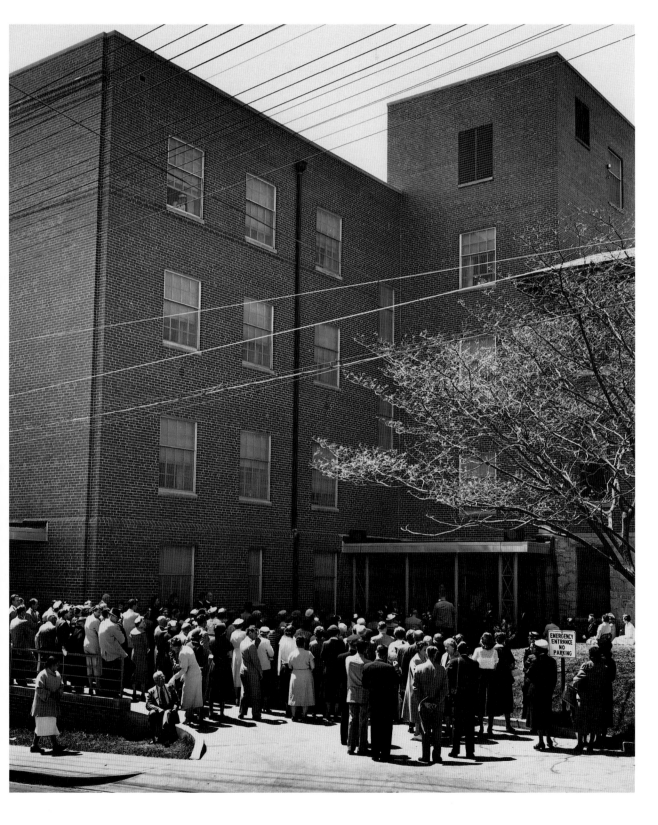

The dedication of the
Baldwin Wing,
May 12, 1955.

ANNE ARUNDEL GENERAL HOSPITAL MET AND SUCCESSFULLY PASSED ONE OF THE MOST CHALLENGING TESTS IN ITS HISTORY LAST NIGHT.

EVENING CAPITAL
February 24, 1956
Reporting on the hospital's response to the
Pennsylvania Railroad train wreck

perature- and humidity-controlled 27-bassinet nursery suite, with stainless steel bassinets, seven incubators for premature babies and a separate room for babies requiring isolation. A new formula and clean-up room had special sterilization and refrigeration equipment.

Emergency and outpatient rooms were revamped and included an air-conditioned operating room, high-speed sterilizer, two-bed recovery room and fracture room. The X-ray department was allotted rooms for the 300- and 500-milliampere units and the fluoroscope, cystoscopic unit and radiation therapy. The "deep therapy" now offered enabled patients to come to Annapolis for treatment rather than having to travel to Baltimore and Washington.

Patient rooms in the Baldwin Wing were decorated in pastels, with tile baths, pantries and waiting rooms on each floor and a large solarium on the third floor. A vacuum system piped oxygen into each room. Communications were improved with a doctor paging system and bedside microphones, allowing patients to talk with nurses at the nurses' station console. Careful planning was evident throughout, even to the doors of patient rooms, which were easily opened by levers rather than the usual door knobs. With adequate medical beds in the new wing, the John B. Rich Building became the pediatric annex. It was connected to the Baldwin Wing with a concrete ramp.

The 1955 hospital was a far cry from its 11-patient predecessor of 50 years before. The total cost of construction, renovation of the old building and equipment came to about $1.75 million. It was paid for with the $600,000 bond issue, $430,000 from the federal government, the Baldwin Foundation grant and the more than $500,000 contributed by citizens and community organizations.

Full utilization of the new hospital's improvements brought a jump in almost all treatments and procedures in 1955. Work in the X-ray department increased more than 71 percent, with some 12,400 exams and treatments logged. Lab work showed a 19 percent increase; the number of operations performed increased by 28 percent to over 2,300, or more than six procedures every day of the year.

There were 5,752 patients admitted during 1955, 857 of them newborns, but for the first time in several years, the occupancy rate fell below 70 percent. There were 7,224 cases treated in the emergency, or accident, room and 2,122 in the orthopedic room, for a total outpatient load of 9,346. The hospital on a whole saw more than 15,000 cases that year. The average hospital stay was seven days.

In 1955, 48 physicians, including four women and four black doctors, constituted the active staff of Anne Arundel General Hospital, with 38 consultants in various specialties. The Board of Managers included members from south county (Bristol, Grennock), Millersville, Arnold, St. Margaret's, Odenton and the Annapolis area. The advisory committee of the board brought particular expertise to the board's discussions and included the chief of the medical staff, an attorney and a clergyman.

Special recognition was given by the *Evening Capital* to county civic organizations that gave equipment or specially designated funds to the new hospital: the Mayo Homemakers Club, Zonta Club, Lions Club, Soroptimists,

Elks and the hospital's own Auxiliary. The Auxiliary planned an enlarged snack bar and gift shop in the renovated older building.

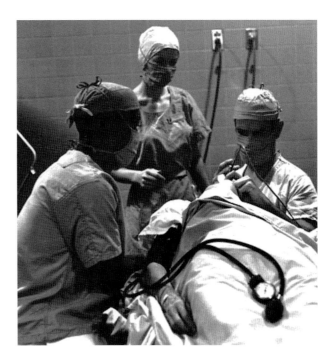

On the evening of February 23, 1956, seven cars of the Pennsylvania Railroad's New York-bound "Embassy" passenger train jumped the tracks near Odenton in one of the county's worst train wrecks. Five passengers were killed and more than 100 injured. Rescue squads from miles around raced to the scene and dispatched their ambulances with the injured to hospitals in Baltimore, Fort Meade and Annapolis. When word of the accident reached Anne Arundel General, hospital administrator Sherrill S. Adams and night supervisor Anne Parkin called in doctors and nurses and set

Green-gowned operating room team, c.1957.

The laboratory in the 1910 (D) building, 1955.

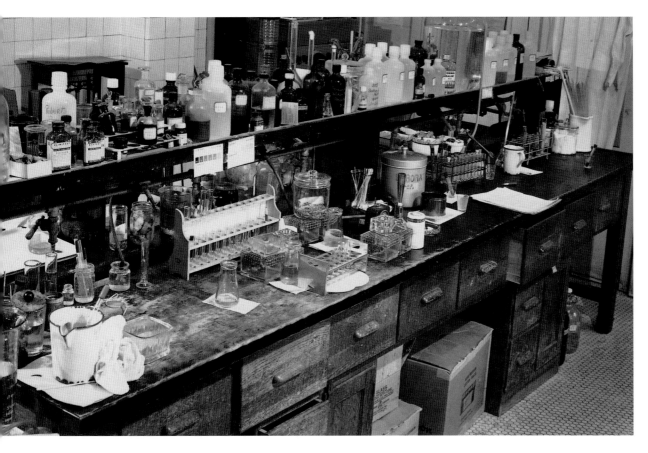

New X-ray machine demonstrated by a nurse and the chief X-ray technician, 1955.

An autoclave and water-distilling equipment, c.1952. On the right is nurse Elaine Donavan, and on the left Florence DeLone, nurse-anesthetist until 1953.

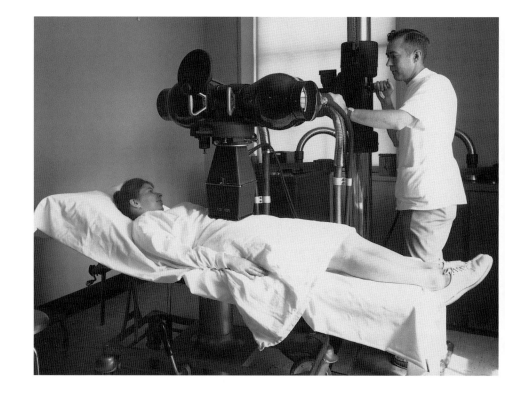

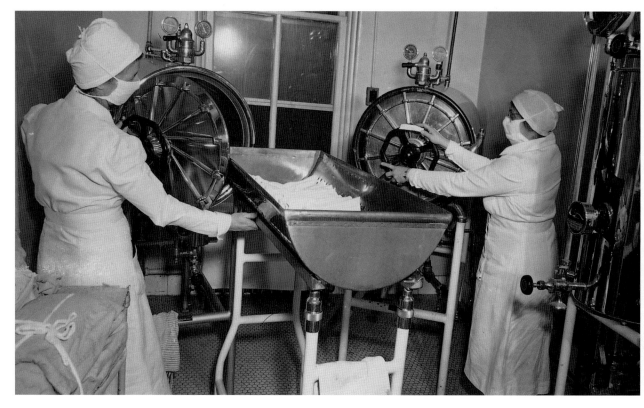

about preparing the emergency room. The first ambulance arrived at 7 p.m. During the night, 20 people, most with severe lacerations or internal injuries, were treated, and 18 were admitted. Some of the staff worked in street clothes, having rushed to the hospital to volunteer for duty as soon as they heard the news. Announcements had been made in movie theaters and other public places. The Washington Red Cross sent blood plasma and the local police helped control the crowd of curious onlookers who milled around outside the emergency room. When it was all over, Mr. Adams praised the staff and the community for their cooperation. The new hospital and its personnel had handled the tragedy efficiently and well.

In his report at the annual meeting of the Annapolis Emergency Hospital Association held in March 1956, President Lynch warned the association that the hospital, even with its enlargement, could not rest on its laurels. The projected population growth for the county, then estimated to reach 195,000 by 1960, made further expansion of the facility necessary to keep pace. Already the board was considering adding 30–40 new beds.

The year 1956 saw the completed renovation of the old building, the remodeling of the pediatric annex, and installation of oxygen supplies and air conditioning throughout. Dental service was added to the list of medical services and Dr. Lyman Milliken was appointed its chief. Dr. Frank M. Shipley, president of the medical staff, reported that the staff continued to hold scientific meetings at which local and visiting speakers could discuss various medical topics. In 1956, he said, 38 percent of the hospital's 167 deaths were autopsied, contributing "immeasurably to the scientific advancement of our hospital community." The hospital admitted 7,144

patients and treated 7,726 cases in the new emergency room.

Graduates of the hospital's nursing school who took the state board exam in 1955 made the highest scores of more than 7,000 practical nurses taking the same exam across the country. Beginning in 1956, only one class was admitted each year in September. The school was commended in February 1957 by the Maryland State Board of Examiners of Nurses and asked to serve as a model for future schools. Of the 50 students who had graduated by March 1957, 37 were employed by the hospital.

Over the next year the hospital and staff adjusted to the demands of what had become a large and sometimes unwieldy institution. Student technical assistants were used in the operating rooms during the summer and four house officers helped with the patient load and emergencies. After the death of Dr. Champo in 1957, staff physicians became responsible for covering the emergency room.

Modern atomic technology stepped into the hospital in 1956 when the lab began using radioisotopes in diagnostic procedures. In 1957, the U.S. Atomic Energy Commission licensed the X-ray department for limited use of two isotopes for treatment of certain diseases.

The hospital's occupancy rate in 1957 had climbed to 74 percent. There were 7,866 patients admitted, 1,266 of them newborns. More than 11,000 cases were treated in the emergency room. With a budget of more than $1 million a year and a patient load close to 20,000 cases, the Anne Arundel General Hospital approached the end of the decade as a substantial business with a critical effect on the lives of the people of Anne Arundel County.

In 1959, hospital administration was a wide open field; I could have gone anywhere. I decided to work here for a few years under Lyman Whittaker, but I fell in love with the area and never left.

The hospital was relatively small when I came. The facilities were not in the best shape; there was no air conditioning in patient rooms. We desegregated restrooms and dining rooms and integrated the employees. It was a culture shock at first!

The hospital didn't have the equipment to be a progressive hospital. Whit's (hospital administrator Lyman C. Whittaker) basic philosophy was, 'If you provide the necessary tools, you'll attract the best doctors.' We sold the board on that philosophy and they were extremely supportive. We were the first hospital in Maryland to get a cineradiography machine to view X-rays, which was a major advancement in radiology. We also looked for the best radiologist—Bob Frazier came to the hospital around 1960. Other specialists followed and in a few years we had a fully qualified staff in all our services. The residents of Anne Arundel County developed confidence in our doctors, and patients stayed here instead of going up to Baltimore.

We were the first non-teaching hospital in the U.S. to have 24-hour coverage in the coronary care unit. A team of seven physicians started the unit and took turns staffing it. *The New England Journal of Medicine* published an article about it, and we received hundreds of requests for information. We also went way out of our way to keep our patients comfortable, with air conditioning, electric beds, television, gourmet meals and many other patient comforts. The patients were really appreciative. We provided more R.N. hours per patient than any hospital in the state.

Plans were underway for the A Building during that time. We thought about leaving downtown then, but it was too expensive. We would have had to sell the hospital to the county or state, but neither was interested. So we made the decision to expand on site instead. The community really supported us, too, and exceeded their $1 million goal in a major fund drive.

Perspective...

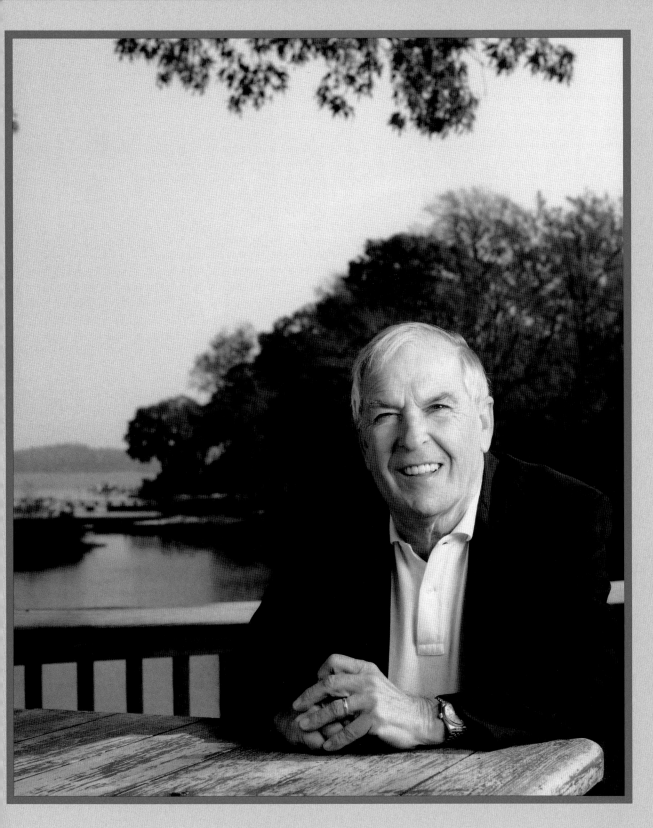

Carl A. "Chuck" Brunetto

Joined hospital as assistant administrator, 1959

Administrator, 1979

CEO of AAGHCS, 1988

President emeritus, 1994

Retired, 1996

The enlarged and modernized Anne Arundel General Hospital attracted young, eager physicians to its staff, doctors who had grown up with the medical advances of the postwar period and who were well trained in the technology still developing. Anne Arundel County and its hospital needed these doctors, as population growth in the county continued, reaching a new high of more than 206,000 residents in 1960. The number of babies born in the hospital almost doubled between 1953 and 1961; lab examinations passed the 100,000-per-year mark in 1960. Between 1957 and 1962, the medical staff of active and courtesy physicians increased by 46 percent, from 57 to 83.

Medical doctors applying each year for privileges within any service of Anne Arundel General Hospital presented their credentials to a committee of the medical staff, which included the chiefs of services. After careful review of the applicants' credentials and qualifications, the committee sent its recommendations to the Board of Managers for final approval.

The credentials committee also acted as a grievance committee, again forwarding its recommendations to the board for action, and with the executive committee of the board, composed a joint committee for the discussion of problems relating to the medical staff.

Although in his report to the Annapolis Emergency Hospital Association in March 1958, Dr. Frank M. Shipley, president of the medical staff, remarked on the "increased understanding and trust between the medical staff and the Board of Managers" during 1957, the authority of the board in granting hospital privileges was challenged in a dispute similar to the one 55 years earlier. Again, a minority of staff physicians took their case to the public and, as in 1903, the hospital association voted to maintain the board's control. The 1958 dispute centered on the long-standing rule prohibiting staff physicians from membership on the board. (The advisability of having physicians on the boards of hospitals in which they practiced was being debated nationally at this time among the members of the Joint Commission on Hospital Accreditation, the American Hospital Association and other groups concerned with hospital management.)

Led by a physician who had been suspended from hospital practice, a small group of interested laymen supported the election of board members whom they considered favorable to staff membership. Also at issue was a proposed change in the association bylaws giving life membership on the board to members who had served five terms as president. The only person to whom this would apply at the time was John B. Rich.

More than 400 people attended the tense annual meeting in the St. Mary's High School gymnasium on March 17, 1958. William J. McWilliams, who had assumed the presidency of the association after the death of Charles B. Lynch less than one week before, carefully controlled the crowd as he refuted charges of the board's "totalitarianism"—a hot word in that Cold War era. Results of the election to the board, announced shortly before midnight, showed that indeed a physician had been elected to the board, but she was Dr. Elizabeth H. Iliff, who was not a member of the hospital medical staff. Of the five candidates proposed by the challenging group, only Dr. Iliff and Sherod L. Earle were added to the board and both of them had previously disavowed in public any connection with or approval of the dissenters. Among the bylaws changes approved by the association

COMING OF AGE
1958 - 1970

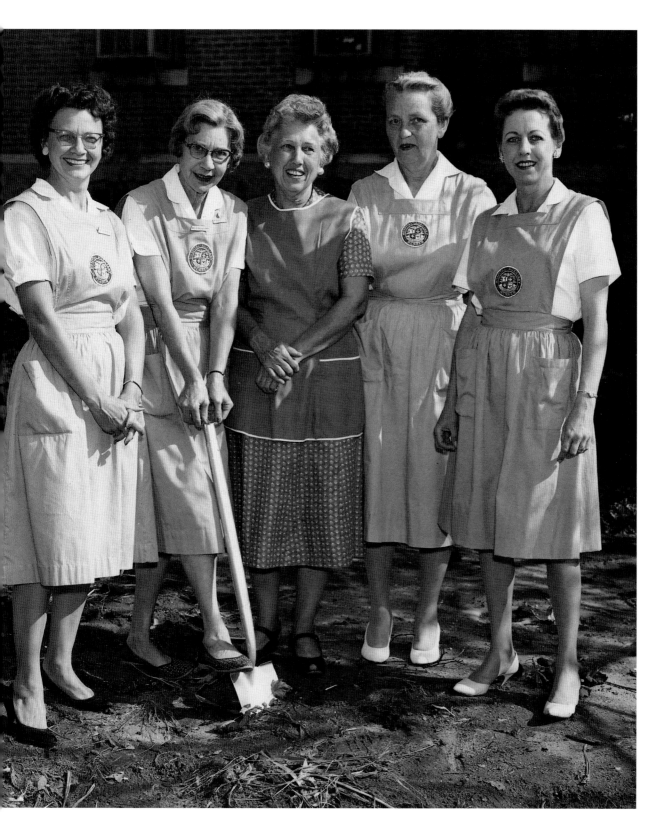

Breaking ground for the expansion of the Hospitality Shop in 1960 were Auxiliary members Mrs. Benjamin T. Myers, Mrs. John Galloway, Mrs. Harry A. Turner, Mrs. Chancey Whitney and Mrs. Mallie A. Griffin.

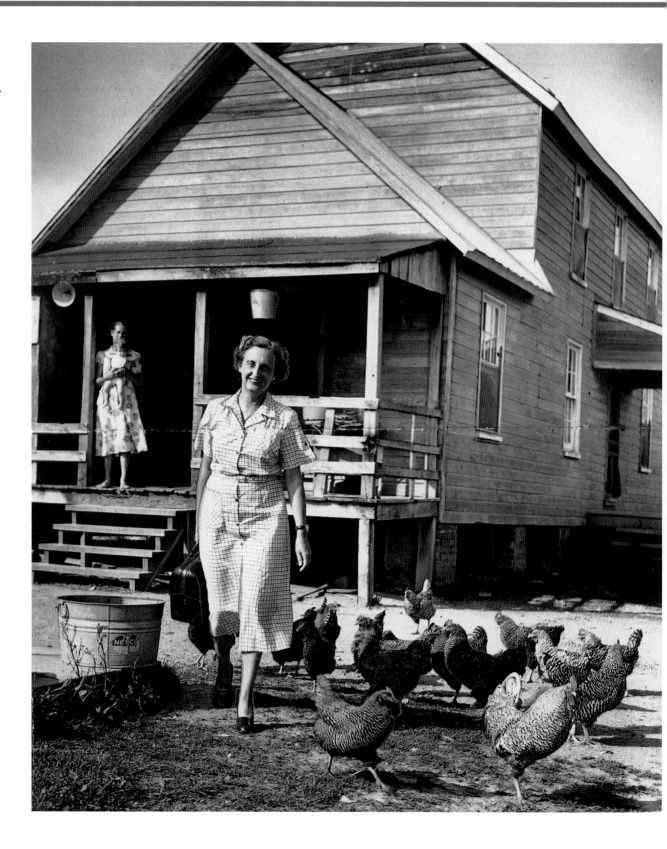

Dr. Emily Wilson made a house call in the 1950s to the Paddy family, who lived on a tenant farm in south county.

was one specifically denying board seats to members of the hospital's medical staff. Also approved was the provision for life membership (to age 75) on the board. (Since then William J. McWilliams, Sherburne B. Walker, McLean S. Welch and Rebecca M. Clatanoff qualified as life members. The bylaw permitting life membership was revoked in 1991.)

In early February 1958, Anne Arundel General Hospital's first professional administrator, Lyman C. Whittaker, reported for duty in the aftermath of a major snowstorm. Slogging through the drifts to the hospital on his first day, Mr. Whittaker found board member McLean S. Welch shoveling snow off the Franklin Street sidewalk at the hospital's entrance. "There was indeed a real hardworking member of the board," said Mr. Whittaker later. "Claney was that kind of man!"

Although the hospital had employed an administrator since 1944, none of the previous men had been formally trained for the position. Upon the death of Sherrill Adams in October 1956, his assistant, Charles T. Smisson, had filled in until Mr. Whittaker's arrival. Mr. Whittaker was the first graduate of the Johns Hopkins School of Public Health hospital administration program and had previously been the assistant administrator at Delaware Memorial Hospital in Wilmington. Carl A. Brunetto joined the staff as assistant administrator in 1959; he had received his Master's degree in hospital administration from Emory University.

One of the new administrator's first tasks was to complete the job of bringing the hospital into full compliance with the standards set by the Joint Commission on the Accreditation of Hospitals. The hospital had received probationary approval from the commission for

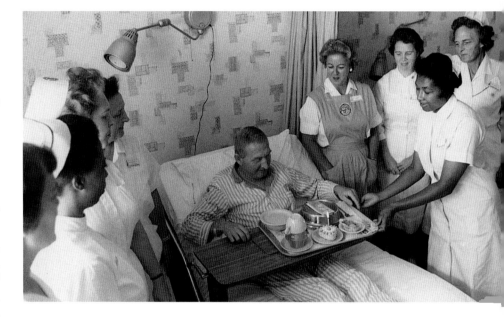

several years, but needed to make a number of improvements to qualify for full, three-year accreditation status.

The Joint Commission, established in 1951 by the American College of Surgeons, the American Medical Association, the American Hospital Association, the American College of Physicians and the Canadian Medical Association, set strict standards for hospitals throughout the country in such areas as physician and staff training and performance, physical plant and equipment, and medical record keeping. On-site inspections and a close review of hospital records by Joint Commission personnel allowed hospitals to see how they measured up in terms of these national standards. Full accreditation by the Joint Commission meant that the hospital delivered quality patient care. Accreditation was to hospitals, said Dr. Frank M. Shipley, what the "sterling" mark was to silver. Anne Arundel General Hospital was granted full accreditation by the Joint Commission for the first time in July 1958. According to Mr.

Patients' birthdays did not go unmarked. Nurses always took the extra step to make patients comfortable and speed recovery.

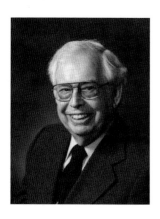

Whittaker, only half the hospitals in the United States and Canada were fully accredited at that time.

That same year, however, the hospital faced a serious problem with staph infections in its orthopedic operating room. Dr. Harold Bohlman, chief of the orthopedic service, canceled open orthopedic surgery, pointing to the air conditioning units as the probable source of the staph contamination. The joint conference committee of the Board of Managers and medical staff initiated a study and improvements were made to the air conditioning in the operating rooms, but the source of the contamination remained unclear. Finally in the fall, after exhaustive testing, further attention was given to air circulation and the problem was solved. Orthopedic surgery resumed under the surgical service and the committee on operating room contamination instituted procedures to ensure that this problem would not recur.

The hospital Auxiliary contributed substantially to the cost of installing air conditioning in the children's annex in the

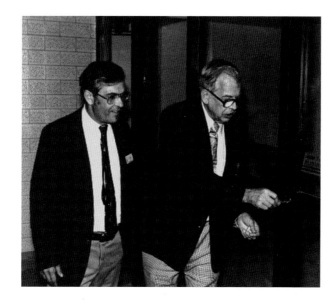

Rich Building in 1958 by holding "A Day at Holly Beach Farm" at the home of Mrs. Henry M. Parr III. By 1959, the Auxiliary was averaging about $25,000 a year in contributions to the hospital and giving about 30,000 hours of volunteer time to its services. Expansions in 1960 gave the Auxiliary additional snack bar and gift shop space.

After more than a half-century of running its own kitchen, the hospital contracted in June 1959 with the A.L. Mathias Co. for food service. The days of donated homemade cakes and preserves, backyard eggs and fresh-killed chickens were over, but hot foods continued to be prepared and cooked in the hospital kitchen by local employees. In 1960, 41 people—dietitians, food supervisors, cooks, kitchen helpers and tray service personnel—served 650 meals each day to patients and staff. "Wake-up Coffee Service" and a selective menu provided patients with choices, and reduced complaints. These and other improvements, detailed in an article by administrators Lyman C. Whittaker and Carl A. Brunetto for *Southern Hospitals* magazine in September 1962, contributed to patient comfort.

The administrators cited new pastel-colored paint and wallpaper, electric beds, phones in semi-private and private rooms, and more room-sized air conditioners as particularly important. The Auxiliary took the hotel-style renovations a step further by offering television service to patients and participating in the Art for Hospitals project, which placed prints and original paintings in the public areas and allowed long-stay patients the opportunity to choose a special picture for their room. The Stork Club, a new waiting room for expectant fathers, opened communication with the delivery room through the use of a two-way speaker system.

Medical improvements during the early 1960s

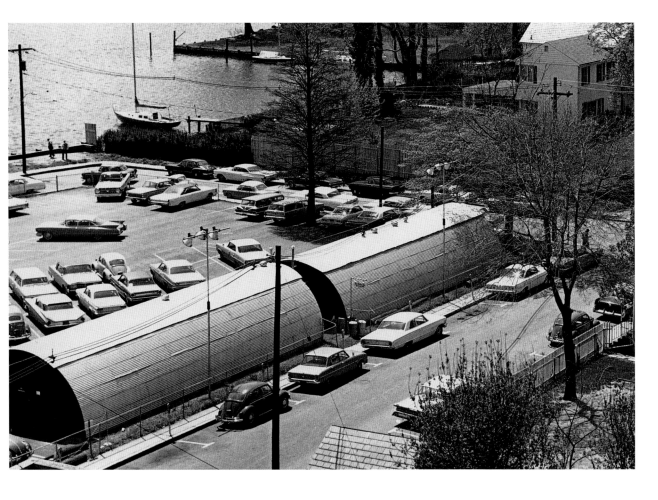

Surplus Navy Quonset huts, pressed into service in the mid-1960s, remained for many years.

included intravenous (IV) and oxygen therapy programs and a patient counseling service, as well as new equipment. The laboratory added a histology section, special chemical lab and an analyzer-computer; the X-ray department gained an X-OMAT and facilities for cineradiography and image amplification. Much of the new equipment was paid for by the Special Equipment Fund, begun with a grant of $13,000 from the Baldwin Foundation and matched by contributions from the Westinghouse Electric Corporation, the Auxiliary and the community.

The Baldwin Foundation also donated $10,000 toward a special study program for physicians and nurses. In 1961, 18 physicians and six nurses used this grant to attend seminars and classes across the country, bringing new knowledge and techniques back to Annapolis.

Training was extended from the hospital to the community with a course for ambulance drivers. Fourteen countywide volunteer companies operated 17 ambulances that brought patients to the hospital's emergency room. Members of the medical staff instituted a 12-lecture course for the volunteer drivers to acquaint them with hospital policies and emergency procedures. The 1962 class drew 21 participants from eight companies.

Looking over the equipment in the new coronary care unit in 1966 are (left to right): McLean S. Welch, president of the Board of Managers; Mrs. James Martin, widow of Dr. Martin, for whom the unit is named; coronary care unit nurse Lynda Kramer and Dr. Gerard Church, chief of medicine.

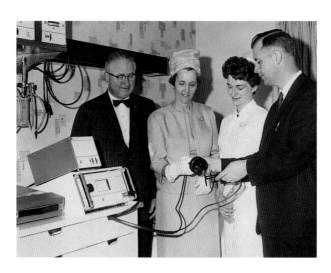

Operating expenses in 1961 passed the $2 million mark, with over 65 percent of the cost of running the hospital paid in salaries to its more than 350 employees. The minimum wage for hospital employees was raised that year to $1 an hour (up from 55 cents per hour in 1959.) Roughly half of the hospital's income came from direct payment of patient fees, the remainder from Blue Cross or other insurance reimbursements and state and county payments for welfare patients. There were always a number of patients not covered by insurance or government funding who could not pay their hospital fees. The resulting deficit was covered, at least in part, by association membership dues and other community contributions.

With occupancy rates climbing steadily above the 75 percent "safe limit" in the early 1960s, the Board of Managers again turned its attention to expansion. Louis Block and Associates, hospital planning consultants, was asked to evaluate Anne Arundel General Hospital's current space problems and recommend solutions. At the annual meeting in March 1963, President McWilliams outlined their conclusions and the board's thinking on the matter.

County growth had not slowed; 1960's population of 206,634 was projected to reach 300,000 in 1970. Planned communities, such as Crofton (1964) and a multitude of smaller developments around Severna Park, would bring more families to the area and demands on the hospital would increase in proportion. Already in 1962, Anne Arundel General Hospital's emergency service load was three times heavier than the average for hospitals of similar size. Worse yet, in comparison with new standards established by the American Hospital Association and the federal government, the existing hospital had a deficit of more than 44,000 square feet to serve its 200 beds.

There was apparently no question in the minds of the board members that substantial enlargement of the hospital's physical plant was in order. The questions were: How big? When? and With what?

The board was thinking seriously about two alternatives: purchasing the rest of the land in the hospital's city block and erecting not just another wing but a new main building at a possible cost of $5 million, or relocating entirely and building a new 300-bed facility outside the city. The estimated cost of this latter plan was $9 million.

At the time that the Annapolis Emergency Hospital Association was pondering these alternatives, ground was broken in 1962 for a new hospital, North Arundel, to serve residents in the northern part of the county. Estimates indicated, however, that even with North Arundel Hospital, the county would still need a larger facility in Annapolis. Then word came of another hospital proposal for the Annapolis area. In February 1963, Dr. Stuart M. Christhilf, Jr., an Annapolis gynecologist and

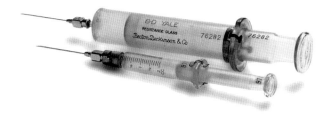

obstetrician, announced plans to build a 75-bed, privately owned Physicians and Surgeons Hospital. The hospital would be located on Riva Road near the recently opened Parole Shopping Center and would admit only private patients for surgical and diagnostic procedures. Amended plans added a separate 50-bed convalescent home. Associated with Dr. Christhilf in this venture was local realtor John W. Steffey.

The Annapolis Emergency Hospital Association feared that the direct effect of this proposed private, proprietary hospital might be to draw from Anne Arundel General Hospital the very patients that kept it vital, reducing it to a municipal charity hospital funded almost entirely by government funds and eventually under government control. Proprietary, profit-making hospitals existed elsewhere in the country, but there were at

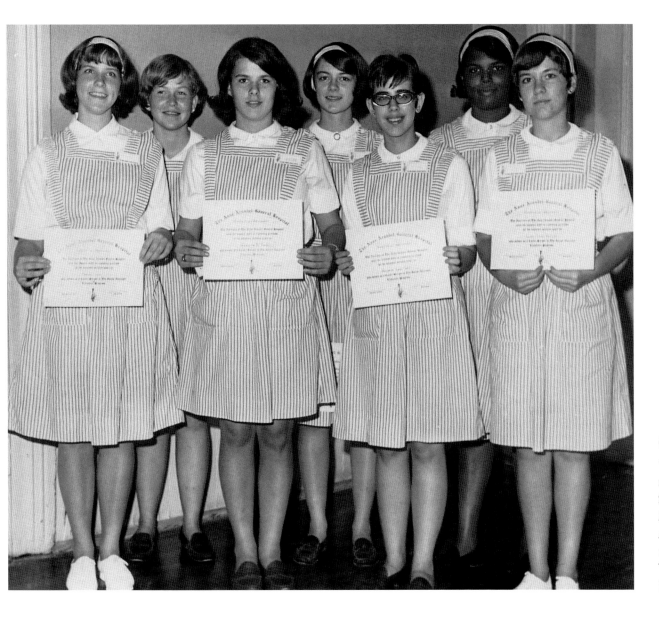

Candy-stripers in 1967. Front (left to right): Denise Law, Suzanne Thorpe, Marjorie Cohn, Susan Armiger. Back (left to right): Ella Grau, Leslie Tilghman, Annie Hillary.

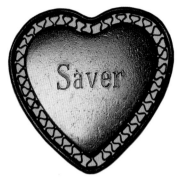

The "saver" pin was given to nurses who resuscitated a patient in the CCU. Four nurses who resuscitated patients in the CCU, wearing their "saver" pins with pride: Effie Slider, Rebecca Mikesell, Lynda G. Kramer, Shirley H. Fuller.

that time no private general hospitals in Maryland. Such a facility was in direct conflict with the mission statement of the Annapolis Emergency Hospital Association, and its membership, as well as the community in general, expressed concern, especially since the proprietors of the new hospital stated that they envisioned both cooperation and an interflow of patients between the two Annapolis hospitals.

Both the State Health Department's Hospital Planning Division and the federal shepherds of the Hill-Burton funds approved the Anne Arundel General Hospital expansion, while neither agency supported North Arundel Hospital or Physicians and Surgeons Hospital. At a special meeting of the Annapolis Emergency Hospital Association in August 1963, President McWilliams outlined the expansion alternatives of Anne Arundel General Hospital and stated that, because the proposed proprietary hospital's mission was incompatible with the nonprofit status of Anne Arundel General Hospital, there could be no cooperation or exchange of patients between the two.

Although many community residents and organizations supported the relocation of Anne Arundel General Hospital to a new, larger site, the board finally accepted the fact that the $9 million cost of such a move was more than the association could realistically expect to raise or borrow. By the fall of 1963, the board had decided to expand on site and examined several plans involving both a new building and renovation of the old ones. At the annual Annapolis Emergency Hospital Association meeting in March, the managers proposed the construction of a nine-story building and some remodeling of the existing structures for an immediate net gain of 54 beds and room for expanded services. To

save money, the top two patient floors of the new building would be left unfinished, holding the potential of an additional 88 beds in the future. The estimated $2,310,000 cost would be covered by federal funds, county bonds, a $1 million state loan and a fund drive to raise $850,000. The tentative schedule called for the construction to be completed in September 1966. Assistant Administrator Carl A. Brunetto was detailed to watch over the planning and construction.

As planning progressed, cost estimates increased by almost $1 million. The community fundraising goal was finally set at $975,000. Again the board turned to Haney and Associates of Massachusetts for assistance with the drive.

McLean S. Welch, president of the board, announced the fundraising campaign in August 1964 at the unveiling of plans for the new building drawn up by architect William H. Metcalf, Jr. of Washington. Overall co-chairmen of the campaign were John B. Melvin and Jerome Lapides, assisted by J. Edward Tyler, Mrs. William B. Clatanoff, Mrs. Buford M. Brown, Mrs. R. Edwin Disharoon, Mrs. Henry M. Murray, Dr. Aris T. Allen, Dr. Manning W. Alden, Harry T. Solomon, Sherod L. Earle, Mrs. Benjamin T. Myers and Honorary Chairman Benjamin Michaelson, Sr.

On September 14, 1964, 1,350 guests from the hospital's service area attended a kick-off community dinner at the National Guard Armory in Annapolis to hear Dr. Morris Fishbein, former president of the American Medical Association; Dr. Barber C. Palmer, president of the medical staff; Mrs. William G. Gideon, president of the Auxiliary; Lyman C. Whittaker and Dr. Manning W. Alden describe the new building and its importance to Anne Arundel County.

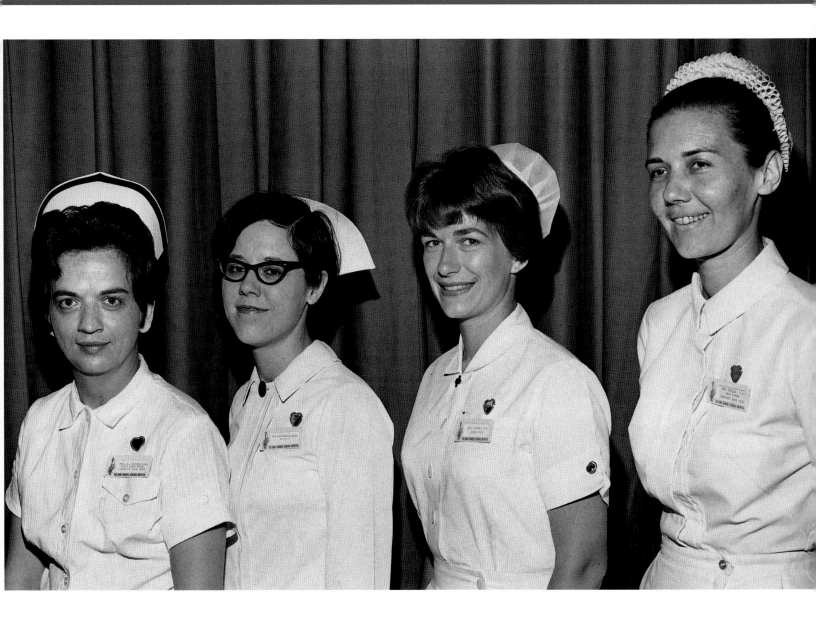

As it had in the past—in 1902 and 1928 and 1949—the community responded to this latest campaign with approval and time and money. Within two months, the building fund was "Over the Top!" with more than $1 million pledged by 6,118 people and organizations. The Auxiliary alone pledged $50,000.

Meanwhile, services in the county's only general hospital continued to increase across the board. The plan for an Annapolis proprietary hospital was dropped and although North Arundel was under construction, it would not open until July 1965. For the moment, county residents would have to make do with the only hospital they had. More than 9,000 of them were admitted to Anne Arundel General Hospital in 1964 and another 20,000 came to the emergency room. There were more than 1,500 babies born in the hospital, 4,000 surgical operations performed, almost 150,000 lab tests made and more than 28,000 X-ray exams and treatments. The daily charge per patient was about $33.

Full racial integration of the hospital took place in the early 1960s, beginning with integration of the staff dining rooms and lavatories in the late 1950s and progressing through the wards to the semi-private rooms. The hospital reflected the general integration of the city's public places during that period and matters went smoothly.

The new wing would be built on land currently occupied by the Nurses' Home, Clothes Box, pediatric unit and the power plant. Finding space to house these functions during construction challenged the administration's imagination. The solution was army surplus trailers for the engineer, housekeeping department and storage; three Navy Quonset huts for the maintenance department and Clothes Box; and the purchase of two houses on Shaw Street for the nursing school and business office. Immediately prior to construction, pediatrics would move to the existing hospital and a temporary boiler plant would be built elsewhere on the property.

In 1966, Medicare Parts A and B became effective, providing people 65 and older with up to 90 days of in-hospital care per illness, outpatient and nursing home care, and physician services. Accreditation by the Joint Commission on Accreditation qualified a hospital to receive federal reimbursement for the care of the elderly. Anne Arundel General Hospital began accepting Medicare patients in July 1966 and slowly, over the remainder of the year, their numbers increased. By the end of the year, almost one-third of the medical-surgical beds held Medicare patients. Many could have been transferred to convalescent

or nursing homes, but such facilities were in short supply. The hospital was inundated with questions, regulations and paperwork. The special care unit was established in 1968 to provide extensive observation and nursing care for elderly and disoriented patients. To help manage its general bookkeeping, the hospital began in 1967 to computerize the business office under the direction of Controller Chad Pierce.

When the Anne Arundel Community College instituted its two-year associate degree nursing program in September 1966, Anne Arundel General Hospital gave these students the opportunity to gain practical experience in a hospital setting. The hospital's own operating room technician training course provided specific instruction to nurses already on the staff to qualify them as assistants to the operating teams. And, under the federal Manpower Development and Training Program, Anne Arundel General Hospital became the first hospital in Maryland to offer a three-week nurse refresher program. Several nurses returned for full- or part-time duty as a result of this course.

The hospital's most outstanding medical event in 1966 was the opening of the coronary care unit (CCU). Named in honor of Dr. James R. Martin, a longtime staff member who died in November 1965, the CCU not only improved the chances for coronary care patients but, over the next few years, brought Anne Arundel General Hospital national recognition and a place in the annals of general hospital medicine.

Special coronary care units in large teaching hospitals with full-time physicians were not uncommon by the mid-1960s, but they were considered out of the reach of a 200-bed community hospital with no designated full-time staff. The physicians and nurses of Anne Arundel General Hospital proved that community hospitals could, in fact, aspire to the improved care offered by the technology of the day and could do it well.

When contributions were given to the medical staff in memory of Dr. Martin, the staff decided to use that money to create a CCU. Under the direction of Dr. Gerard Church and with the cooperation of the board and the administration, two semi-private rooms in the Baldwin Wing were converted to one large four-bed room. Monitoring equipment with a visual alarm next to each bed displayed the patient's electrocardiogram, and a "crash cart," with a direct-current defib-

rillator, oscilloscope and electrocardiographic recorder, was located nearby. Another crash cart was placed in the emergency room. Setting up the physical unit was fairly easily accomplished and was done at a cost of only about $10,000. Staffing it was another matter.

The physicians involved—Drs. Frank M. Shipley, Gerard Church, Richard N. Peeler, Richard S. Hochman, Charles W. Kinzer, Edward S. Beck and, later, Peter F. Verkouw, Robert O. Biern and Ray M. Smith—all had extensive private practices. But each was willing to take a three-day stint as CCU physician, during which time he assumed total responsibility for the care of unit patients. He could maintain his private practice, but his

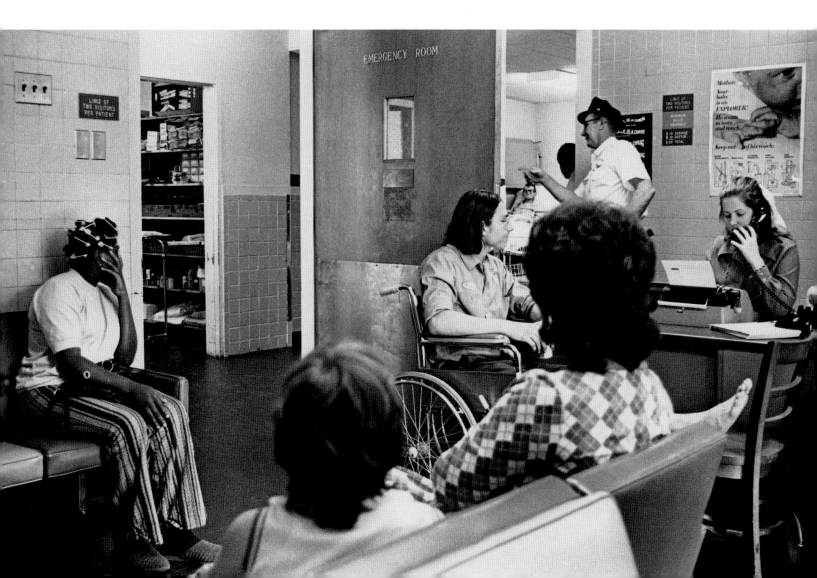

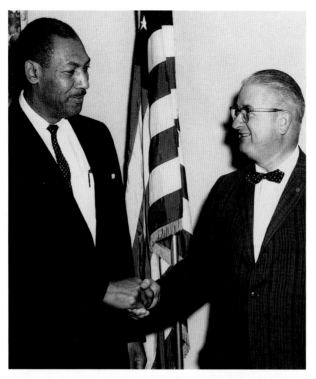

Dr. Aris T. Allen (left) receives congratulations from McLean S. Welch, president of the Board of Managers, on the success of his fundraising efforts.

Over the Top! with more than $1 million in community pledges, November 1964.

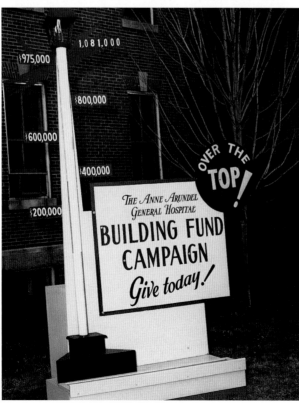

duty in the CCU took precedence and he had to remain within a few minutes of the hospital.

The full-time CCU staff was drawn from the hospital's registered nurses, offering them patient care responsibilities previously denied nurses. Lynda G. Kramer, Shirley H. Fuller, Rebbeca Mikesell and Effie Slider, R.N.s on the hospital staff, volunteered quickly for CCU duty. They, and the other nurses in the program over time, trained for two months, with lectures by staff physicians, reading assignments and practice. At first, the nurses were limited in their treatment of cardiac arrest, but after a few months they were allowed to use the defibrillator and, eventually, to give intravenous drugs in certain emergency situations. Licensed practical nurses and nurses aides assisted the R.N.s in full-time coverage and were taught to recognize arrhythmias.

Within months, it was apparent that the CCU was living up to its promise—deaths resulting from acute myocardial infarction dropped by half. After three years and some 300 CCU patients, the overall death rate was 55, or 18 percent. Dr. Church, Mrs. Kramer and others on the team wrote papers and delivered lectures on the Anne Arundel General Hospital CCU, stressing that with properly trained nurses and the sacrifices of willing physicians, community hospitals like Anne Arundel General Hospital could offer this lifesaving benefit to their patients. Physicians came from across the country to ask questions and examine the program. Presentations to regional and annual meetings of the American College of Physicians and a subsequent article by Dr. Church and Dr. Biern published in *The New England Journal of Medicine* in 1969 drew international attention.

The success of the CCU prompted the

medical staff, under Chief of Surgery J. Fred Hawkins and Chief of Anesthesiology Jack Lyons, to establish an intensive care unit in 1967 for the supervision and treatment of other critically ill patients. Again, specially trained nurses provided concentrated around-the-clock care.

By the late 1960s, the Auxiliary was such an integral part of hospital life that no one could imagine the building without the cheerful cherry-pink-clad volunteers. More than half the 600 members gave time weekly to Auxiliary activities, almost 45,000 hours in 1965 alone. Among the more popular patient services were the "pinky puppets" for children and the baby picture service for new mothers. In 1967, the Auxiliary expanded its television rental service into a closed circuit broadcasting operation with WPPG, Channel 6. Channel 6 carried programs of interest to the patients ("Care for Your Baby," "Hobby Lobby") throughout the day, as well as in-service classes for L.P.N.s and the local afternoon soap opera, "Visit-Vision," which allowed children too young to visit in their parents' rooms to talk with them on the phone from the lobby while their parents (and anyone else) tuned in on their antics via the television.

The Auxiliary's junior volunteer program, begun in the late 1950s, gave teenage girls an opportunity to learn about patient care and volunteering. Called "candy-stripers" because of their pink-and-white-striped pinafores, girls ages 15 to 20 could choose to work as junior nurses' aides and assist with patient care or as junior Auxiliary volunteers and help with volunteer activities. The latter were particularly welcome in the children's playroom. The girls attended preparatory classes and agreed to give at least 100 volunteer hours to the hospital during their summer vacation. Second-year nursing volunteers became "pinkies," with cherry-pink pinafores. They often worked throughout the year and many went on to nursing school. By the late 1960s, candy-stripers and pinkies were giving thousands of hours each year to the hospital.

Volunteer services were only one factor of the Auxiliary's commitment to the hospital. Another important activity was raising money for the general operation of the hospital or for special projects such as the nurses' library or, in the late 1960s, to fulfill pledges of $150,000 to the building fund for the new A wing. In addition to hospital-based money-makers such as the Clothes Box or Hospitality Shop, each year the Auxiliary held large, lucrative events. Some of these, such as the symphony concerts, enriched the cultural life of the county. Others were pleasant social events—the fashion shows and, beginning in 1966, the Pink Lady Ball and A Day at Laurel Raceway. Ever since, the Pink Lady Ball has drawn a sell-out crowd of hospital and community couples. Carrying the hospital's message to the community and involving local individuals and businesses in its work are important adjuncts of the Auxiliary's social and cultural activities.

Throughout 1968 and 1969, construction of the new building placed additional strains on the hospital's facilities and staff. Complaints about the food service led to the more popular four-meal plan and the nursing administration was reorganized to a unit manager system. Outside the hospital, workers of the Consolidated Engineering Company of Baltimore created an ever-expanding maze of concrete and steel, ladders and scaffolds. Patients were spared the deep monotonous thumps of pile drivers because Consolidated used a giant drill to dig holes for the concrete supports of the new

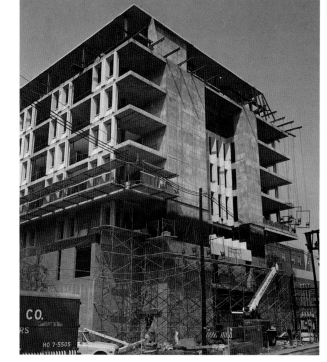

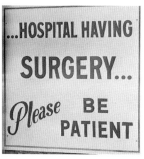

The South (A) Building under construction in September 1968.

operating suite with its recovery room and nine-bed intensive care unit, and the emergency services area, opening also from Cathedral Street, spread across the remainder of the first floors of the South and Baldwin buildings to encompass a large, well-designed complex of services for both in- and outpatient surgery and treatment. The second, third and fourth floors would accommodate pediatric, teenage and adult patients—the latter separated, with medical patients on the third floor and surgical on the fourth. Rooms were located around a central nursing station and utility area, and two "Day Rooms," or visiting areas, on each floor overlooked Franklin Street and Spa Creek. The fifth and sixth floors, with the capacity for 88 beds, were left unfinished. Above them, the top two floors, hidden by the slate mansard roof, housed equipment for high pressure steam heat and central air conditioning.

The new building would add 125 beds immediately and allow further expansion when necessary. The hospital managers had learned the lessons of earlier expansions and the county's population growth over the last 30 years. This time they figured to plan ahead. Equally important, the new $6.5 million building added space for essential services and for the new diagnostic and treatment machinery becoming so much a part of patient care. It also provided for mechanized supply and communications systems to speed and simplify the overall operation of the hospital.

Dedication ceremonies on November 22, 1969, were conducted on the uncompleted fifth floor by Sherburne B. Walker, president of the Board of Managers. The Rev. James P. Madison of St. Anne's and the Rev. Francis R. Salman of St. Mary's offered the invocation and benediction. Speakers included Dr. Richard N. Peeler, president of the medical

structure, but there was noise and dust and lots of activity to watch from the windows.

Variously known as the South Building or A Building, because its rooms carry the A designation, Anne Arundel General Hospital's new wing rose during 1969 to its full height of nine stories. The ground floor, visible only from the low south and east sides of the property, would house service areas: a new kitchen, cafeteria and dining room, meeting rooms, a central service area, receiving dock, electrical substation and a new pharmacy.

The first floor offered a street-level entrance and lobby with a new information desk, to be staffed largely by Auxiliary volunteers, and admitting, computer and business offices. The laboratory, four times larger than the previous one and operated by Arundel Pathology Laboratory, the radiology department, the

... A DRAMATIC STEP FORWARD IN FACILITIES AND SERVICE FOR AN
INSTITUTION THAT HAS ALWAYS BEEN FAMOUS FOR BOTH.

ANNE ARUNDEL TIMES
November 20, 1969

staff; Mrs. John B. Wright, president of the Auxiliary; and Lyman C. Whittaker, administrator. There were concerts by the Naval Academy Band and the Annapolis Choral Society. After the ceremonies, visitors toured the new building, led by members of the Auxiliary, and talked with beaming hospital personnel about the new facilities and equipment.

McLean S. "Claney" Welch, who had devoted so much effort to the realization of this moment, watched the ceremonies on closed circuit television from his bed in the hospital. He died just a few months later.

After more than seven years of planning and construction, the modern Anne Arundel General Hospital inspired the pride and confidence of its community. Annapolis and Anne Arundel County looked forward to a new era in health care.

The dedication of the South (A) Building took place on the unfinished fifth floor. The Annapolis Choral Society participated in the ceremonies.

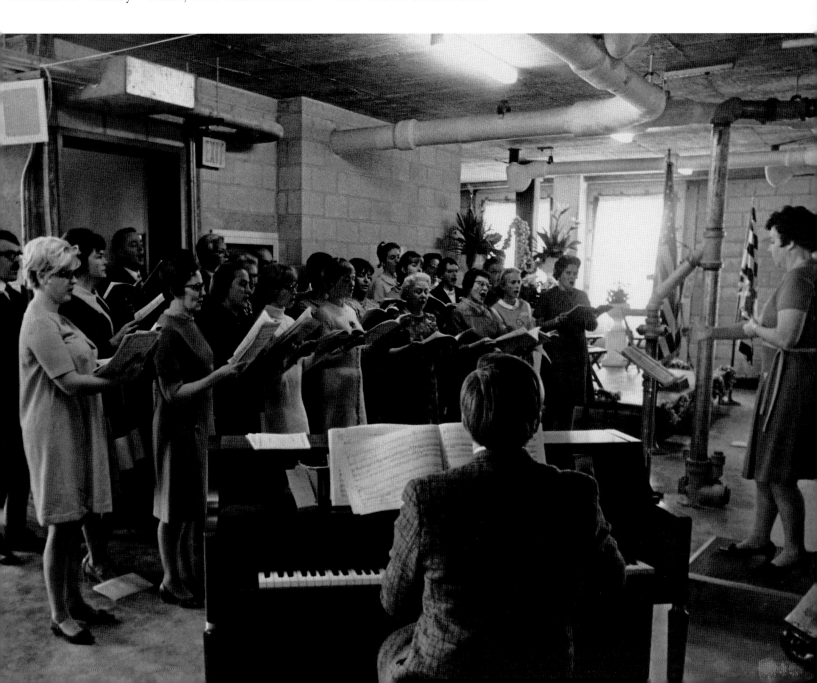

finished my residency at Johns Hopkins and began practice in Annapolis in 1957. There were only 35 doctors on the medical staff; you could have a cocktail party at home and invite everybody!

I charged $4 for an office visit and $8 for a house call. That first year I grossed $16,000. One year later, I joined up with Frank Shipley and we bought some property at 121 Cathedral Street and set up practice there.

There were only a few generalists in town, so we saw everything. Patients didn't have to be so sick to go in the hospital then. A patient who had a heart attack would stay in the hospital for 4-6 weeks, with 3 weeks of total immobility. An appendectomy patient would stay 7-10 days. We even sometimes admitted patients for executive physicals.

Starting in the late 1960s, a lot of new people joined the medical staff. In most cases, individual practices recruited new members. We were able to attract top doctors, because we were near Baltimore and Washington, where a lot had trained. Plus, Annapolis is such a nice environment. They could see that the hospital was expanding rapidly, too. We opened the A Building, renovated the Baldwin Wing, expanded emergency services and maternity services and added psychiatric services. And, of course, there was the parking garage!

These new doctors brought with them new skills and new techniques. All the doctors worked together to find inventive ways to expand hospital services. We needed a CAT scanner, so the neurologists rented space from the hospital, leased equipment and set up a private service. We wanted to add pulmonary function testing, so we found some space in the hospital, purchased equipment and then recruited a pulmonologist to head the lab. Nuclear medicine was another saga. We had to convince the Board of Managers that it was necessary, show that it would pay for itself and then the board finally approved it.

Persistence paid off. We figured out a way around things and removed stumbling blocks. Whit [hospital administrator Lyman Whittaker] worked with us, but our agendas were not always the same. There was always some future goal in mind.

Perspective...

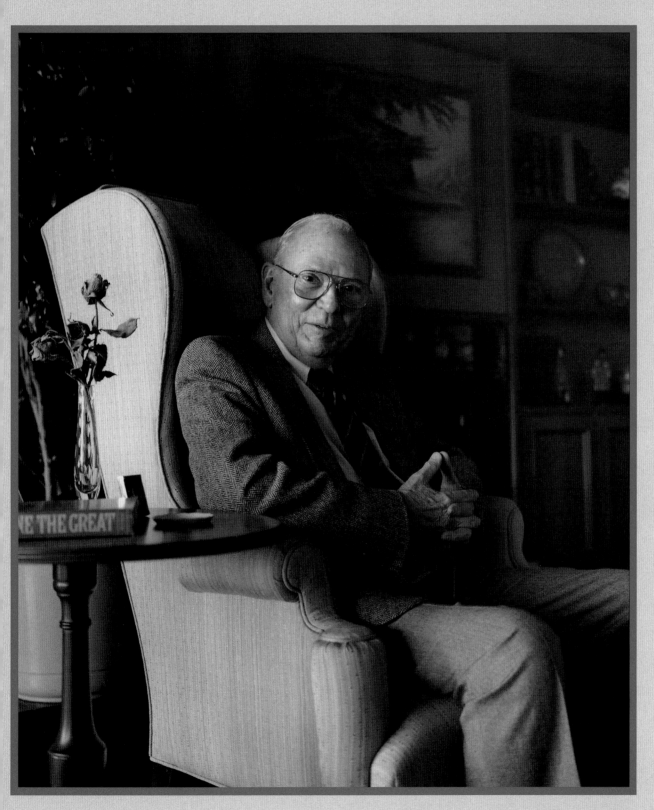

Dr. Richard N. Peeler

Established internal medicine practice, 1957

Medical staff president, 1969-1971

Chief epidemiologist, 1994-1999

Father of Dr. Mark O. Peeler, AAMC vascular surgeon

The 1970 census figures showed Anne Arundel County's population nearing the 300,000 mark—an increase of 30 percent over 1960, 60 percent over 1950 and more than three times the 1940 figure. Ten percent of the county's 1970 residents lived in Annapolis and, after a period of neglect exacerbated by the opening of the Parole Shopping Center, the downtown was beginning to renew itself. Tourists tramped the streets in the wake of Historic Annapolis guides.

Population growth intensified north of the Severn and spread from Annapolis south across the South River. Crofton was a grand success. Everywhere it seemed that fields were growing houses; and roads, schools and the county's hospitals were hard pressed to accommodate the changes. Home rule in Anne Arundel County under the charter government in 1965 replaced the county commissioners with a county council, which tried to get control of population growth and the demand for public services.

The newly enlarged Anne Arundel General Hospital was ready for the challenge. As the staff adjusted to the new building and the reorganization it required, there were still sick patients to care for—27,000 of them sought emergency treatment in 1970.

Through the difficult days of 1970, as problems surfaced and were solved, there were clear bright spots: the school for practical nurses again achieved accreditation, the special care unit was moved and enlarged to 11 beds, a new medical and nursing library was planned, and the Hospitality Shop expanded. The computer center, with its first IBM machine, became a model for other hospitals in the state, including the University Medical Centers in Baltimore. The new

Hydrasposal dry-waste disposal system, a prototype developed by AMSCO Equipment Manufacturers, neatly and cleanly took care of the 16 pounds of waste per patient each day and reduced the amount of trash to be disposed of by 80 percent.

In the late spring, a group of private physicians contracted to provide full-time coverage for the emergency department. This arrangement was similar to that in effect for the clinical laboratory since 1967. The demands on both services made it impossible to staff them with physicians who had a private practice outside the hospital. Staff physicians continued as on-call consultants for these services as well as for X-ray and anesthesiology, the CCU and ICU. Dr. Richard N. Peeler, president of the medical staff, estimated these on-call hours in 1970 as well in excess of 122,000. In addition to on-call consultation, the hospital's staff physicians, comprising 14 general practitioners, 81 specialists and 12 dentists, gave freely of their time to serve on medical staff and specific service committees, teach in-house continuing education classes and offer informed consultations and instruction. A number of the local doctors held teaching positions or privileges at the large hospitals in Baltimore and Washington, and these contacts helped strengthen their experience and commitment to continued education.

The medical audit committee, instituted in 1971, added the power of computerized analysis to the continuing evaluation of each physician's performance, comparing cases with local and national norms. In 1972, staff physicians began meeting regularly by department to share the latest innovations in treatments for their specialties.

The pulmonary function (1971) and nuclear

Nurse Kitty Sharkey cared for thousands of new county residents during her years in the nursery.

102

A Thoroughly Modern
Hospital *1970 - 1979*

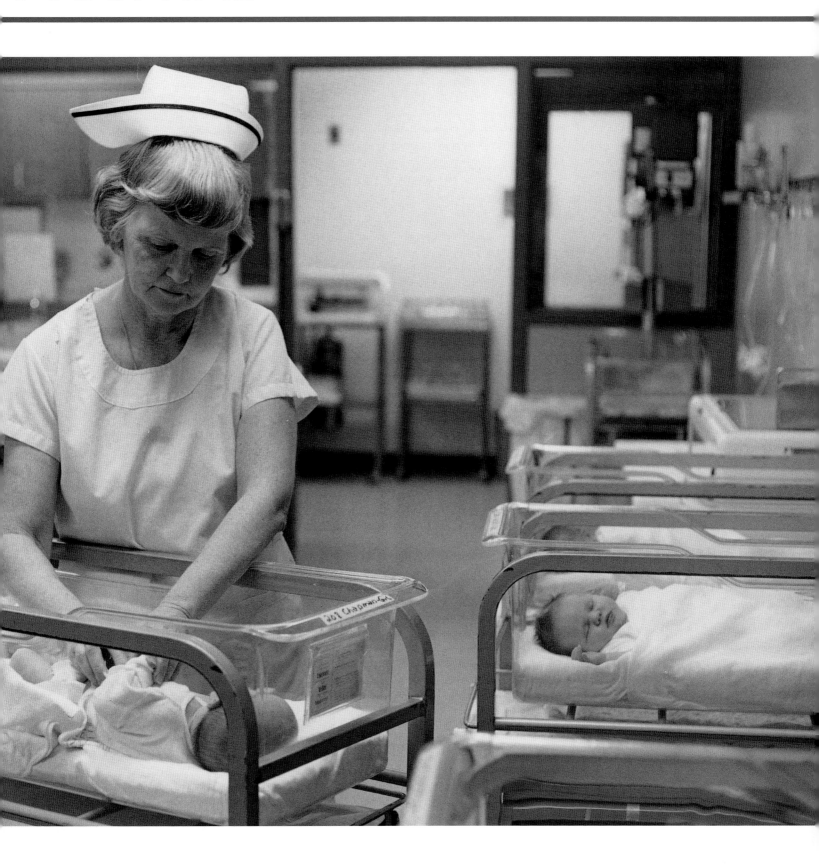

The hospital's engineering department, headquartered in a Quonset hut, was capable of minor repairs or major renovations.

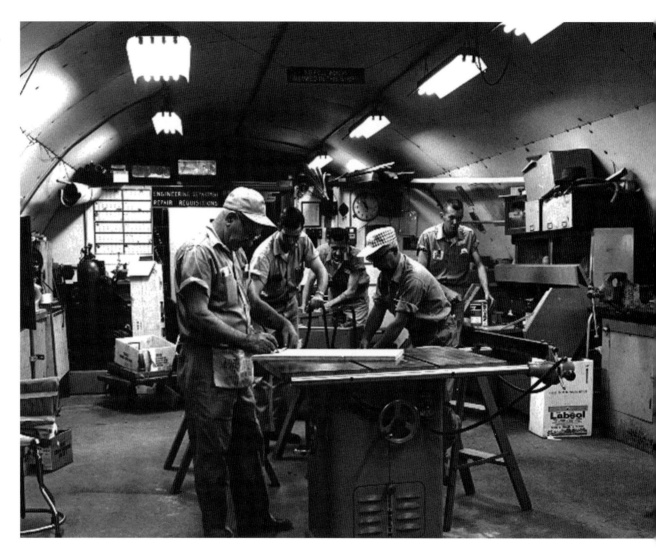

medicine (1973) services illustrate the two general methods by which the hospital's medical services have been expanded over the years. In the first instance, Dr. R. Bruce Helmly arrived in Annapolis already well trained in his subspecialty and initiated the first artificial ventilation program in 1970 and the pulmonary function laboratory in 1971. That year, he became the first chief of the pulmonary function service. In the second instance, that of nuclear medicine, the impetus came from within and required three years of study and discussion before becoming a reality. In 1970, Dr. Peeler, then president of the medical staff, sent questionnaires to 35 community hospitals in Maryland and Northern Virginia requesting information on their radioisotope scanning programs. He also contacted doctors on the Anne Arundel General Hospital staff for statistics on the need within their practices for scanning procedures. Dr. Henry N. Wagner, chief of the division of nuclear medicine at Johns Hopkins, assisted in presentations to the staff and

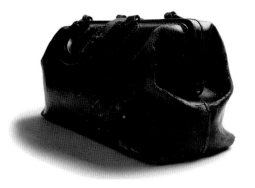

Board of Managers. Of the hospitals surveyed, 29 had scanning facilities, or would have them in 1971, and most were showing a financial, as well as a medical, profit. With the continued assistance of Dr. Wagner and the approval of the staff and board, the hospital assembled the equipment and personnel to initiate the service and bring Anne Arundel General into the era of modern imaging.

Whether the result of fortunate circumstances or long-range planning, the introduction of a new medical service has always depended upon the approval of the staff and board and the availability of trained personnel, as well as the necessary equipment.

In 1971, Charles T. Smisson, "Charlie" to almost everyone, retired after 23 years as assistant administrator. His retirement, plus the loss of two others on the administrative staff and increasing government paperwork, prompted the hiring of a full-time personnel director and the appointment of long-time nursing supervisor Mrs. Alice Banks as assistant administrator, with additional responsibilities for professional services, such as IV therapy, electrocardiogram, inhalation therapy and pulmonary function, and physical therapy. A survey by the planning committee of the board drew recommendations from the medical board for the improvement of the emergency service and the labor and delivery facility. In addition to the newborn nursery, construction for which began in 1971, it appeared that even more building would be required.

Also in the planning stages was a larger parking lot for hospital personnel and visitors. The hospital's 600 or so employees, 100 physicians and the hundreds of daily Auxiliary volunteers and visitors required some place to leave their vehicles. Street parking was not the answer, nor was the lot created behind the houses on Shaw Street that the hospital had been buying over the previous few years. There was talk of a garage.

Sidewalk superintendents had a field day in the spring of 1971 when four of the Shaw Street houses were jacked up, ready to be moved to barges in Spa Creek and floated up to the boat ramp at Truxton Park. Local residents, curious visitors, small children and dogs checked on the big event daily, and many of them even went over to the park to watch the first of these substantial buildings trucked up the bank and over to the farm of Dr. and Mrs. Walter E. Landmesser, Jr., off Hilltop Lane. Against all odds and the prediction of head-shaking skeptics, the first stages of the procedure went smoothly. Then disaster! A house-heavy barge sank at the end of Shaw Street, flooding its cargo. Dr. Landmesser refused to abandon the idea, however, and the remaining houses were moved intact. They stand today on Milkshake Lane.

The newborn nursery, built on the former sun porch of the Baldwin Wing, featured a separate public observation area and was the first in the state to receive approval under the new Maryland Health Department standards. It became the model for other hospitals, and architects came to see the latest concepts in newborn care realized by a community hospital.

Changes in the public's attitude toward birthing prompted changes in the hospital's delivery and maternal care facilities. Prospective mothers and fathers wanted to participate fully and together in the delivery of their babies. In 1972, a patient pleaded for her husband's presence during labor and was allowed to have him stay with her in a room

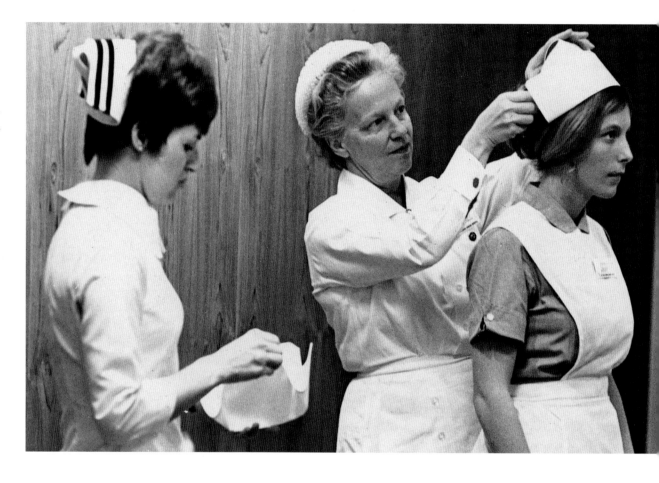

removed from the labor and delivery suite; in 1974, they were welcomed into the labor room together for the birth of their second child. The prepared childbirth program, instituted in 1973 by obstetricians and the nursing coordinator for maternal and child health, offered prospective parents a six-week training in natural childbirth techniques.

The success of the first coronary care unit (CCU) prompted its expansion to an eight-bed unit in 1972. Gifts in memory of Buford M. Brown, who died in 1966, and from a benefit dinner sponsored by Milton Bluefeld, whose life was saved in the CCU in 1971, were dedicated to the improvements. The hospital's maintenance department handled

the renovation, saving hundreds of thousands of dollars in construction costs. The new CCU incorporated the most modern patient care facilities and added a visitors' waiting room.

The contrast between the bright, open, ultra-modern South Building and the cramped, well-used Baldwin Wing, which had itself seemed so modern only 15 years before, struck everyone as a problem. Improved materials for fireproofing, new methods of climate control, innovations in room design and patient-nurse communications—all had been incorporated into the construction of the South Building but were lacking in the Baldwin Wing. The Board of Managers, administrators, medical staff and patients realized that renovation of the old building was in order. Fund drives in 1972 and 1973 made it possible to replace the old windows with thermal pane glass and install under-window heating and cooling units. New corridor ceilings and lights and additional cosmetic improvements helped to make the older wing more cheerful. The Auxiliary paid for new color television sets for all Baldwin rooms. A massive move in 1973 to align the main services (ob/gyn, pediatrics, medical and surgical) on the same floors in both buildings allowed for more convenient access to patients and treatment centers.

After 13 years of contracting with major food service suppliers for operation of the meal program, the hospital returned to in-house food service in 1972. Patients were still served four meals a day with selective menus and the overall costs were reduced.

The hospital's budget was pressed to keep pace with innovations in medical machinery. Each item carried a price tag that would have seemed outrageous 20 years before; but then these items had not been available in the 1950s: cryosurgical equipment for surgical procedures at $3,000, a new blood-gas analyzer at $3,800, a Seiman's radiographic machine at $150,000.

By 1973, the hospital's annual budget was close to $7 million. Because Blue Cross, Medicare and Medicaid reimbursements were considerably less than the actual cost of services and because there were always uncollectible patient bills, the hospital generally showed a deficit that had to be covered through contributions, non-care fees and the income from various gifts and endowments. Some 62 percent of the budget went to direct patient services, including nursing care and support services, food, laundry, etc. The

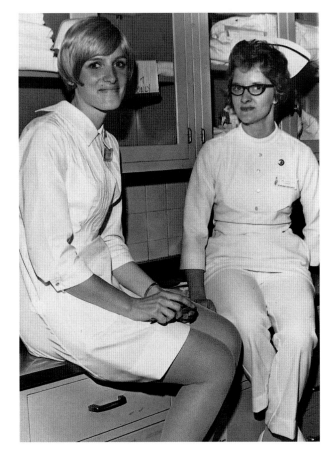

Nurse Kathy Anderson wore the traditional dress in a 1970 fashion show, but Lueva Shuman chose a new pants suit. Clothing was not the only change for nurses in the 1970s.

remaining 38 percent was divided among housekeeping and maintenance (10 percent), depreciation and interest on loans (8 percent), administration expenses, including employee benefits (7 percent) and fiscal and general expenses (13 percent). The hospital admitted 10,573 patients in 1973 and treated another 31,141 through the emergency service—roughly 25 percent more than the number of patients treated in 1968, before the opening of the South Building.

Just over three years after the opening of the South Building, the board again turned to the community for money to build a new wing on the north side of the hospital complex. The three-story addition would lie parallel to the 1928 wing between the original building and the Baldwin Wing and abut Cathedral Street. It would house an expanded emergency services department on the first floor, with entrances from the street for ambulances and patients, and an enlarged labor and delivery suite on the second floor adjacent to the newborn nursery and maternity rooms. The third floor would allow space for the growing X-ray, nuclear medicine, physical therapy and pulmonary function departments. A third of the estimated $3 million cost would go to equipment. Board President Walker and planning committee chairman Rebecca M. Clatanoff were co-chairmen of the fundraising campaign.

In granting its approval for the required variance in March 1973, the city's zoning appeals board specified that the hospital must also begin a parking garage within two years. This was no surprise; parking problems throughout the city provoked columns of letters to the editors of the *Evening Capital.*

Local organizations, such as the Lions Club, which donated $25,000 in June 1973, as well as businesses and individuals again rallied to the hospital's support. The Auxiliary pledged $500,000. Architect Roger L. Pompei of Arlington drew up plans for the building and matters appeared to be going smoothly. However, in February 1974, the board had its first skirmish with the city's new Historic District Commission (HDC).

The designation of downtown Annapolis as a Historic District was added to the city code in 1957. Twelve years later, a city-wide referendum put teeth in the ordinance by setting up the HDC and giving it the power of review and approval for building plans within the historic district before a building permit could be issued.

The HDC, backed by representatives of Historic Annapolis, Inc. and the Ward One Association, requested modification of the new wing's facade. Hospital officials stressed that delays in the construction schedule would add to the cost and postpone completion of the much-needed building. As it turned out, the delay lasted only a few weeks, the modified facade was approved in early March and construction plans continued—after the zoning variance that had expired during the HDC problem was renewed. The hospital's next meeting with the HDC would not be resolved so easily.

The new emergency services area of the $4.2 million Cathedral Street wing opened in June 1976 with more than four times the space of the previous one. Nine treatment rooms, a triage area, facilities for emergency dental and eye treatment, and a large waiting room promised long-awaited improvement in the logistics of emergency patient management. Additional space, following renovation of the existing emergency room, would contain a coronary care unit, operating room and other treatment and supply areas.

For most of its life as an institution, the Anne Arundel General Hospital, along with other community hospitals, stood delicately balanced between its Board of Managers, its administration and its medical staff. Administrator Whittaker often referred to this relationship as a "three-legged stool." Over the years, the three groups had learned to work together toward their common goal—the best possible care and treatment of the hospital's patients. By the mid-1970s, a fourth body emerged as a controlling force in hospitals across the country—government, in all its forms. Federal, state and local governments began to play an increasingly impor-

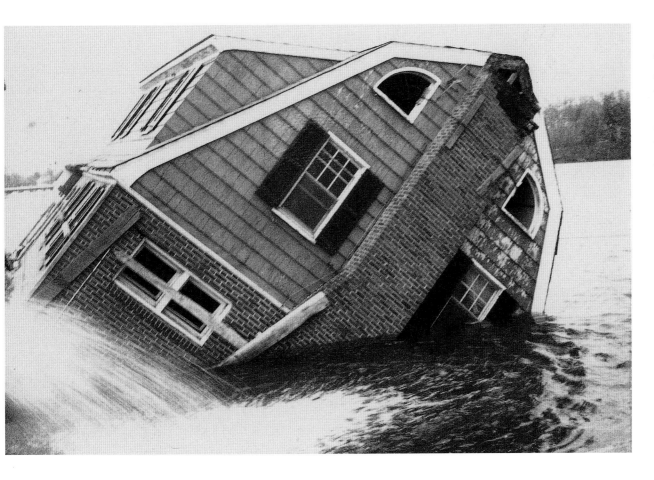

In the spring of 1971, four Shaw Street houses owned by the hospital were jacked up and moved to barges at the end of the street. They were to be floated across Spa Creek and moved to Milkshake Lane, their new home. One of the barges sank with its cargo aboard, but the others were transported without incident.

tant role in both the day-to-day life of the hospital and in its long-range planning processes. State, county and city financing had always been critical to Anne Arundel General Hospital's operation, but the governmental participation now emerging went far beyond direct financial assistance.

Anne Arundel General Hospital felt the effects of government control on all levels, from the Annapolis Historic District Commission to the Maryland Regional Planning Council, the Maryland Health Services Cost Review Commission and the National Labor Relations Board. The hospital's original three entities could no longer simply balance each other; they now had to work together with, or

against, a much larger system, a bureaucracy not of their making.

There were several simultaneous issues of dispute between the entities of this new four-legged stool during the mid- and late 1970s: the completion and opening of the unfinished two floors of the South Building, the question of a nurses' union, the operation of a CAT scanner and the construction of a parking garage. Eventually all were resolved, but in each case the experience took its toll on the hospital board and staff and, in at least one case, on the community as well.

The need for utilizing the two extra floors sitting empty in the South Building was

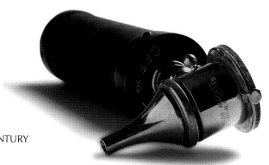

EAR, NOSE AND THROAT APPLIANCE, C.MID-20TH CENTURY
Courtesy of Dr. Michael S. Epstein

obvious to all by 1975. Although the average hospital stay was cut to just 6.4 days in 1974, there were long waits for non-emergency admissions. Opening the two floors meant providing as well all the ancillary services these 88 or so patients and their visitors and caretakers would need. A freeze by the Regional Planning Council on the addition of new beds to hospitals in the Baltimore area held up the plans for a year. Permission was granted in 1976 with the stipulation that a portion of the new beds be used for the care of psychiatric patients.

Establishment of the psychiatric service in 1977 reflected changes in medical thinking regarding the treatment of the mentally ill. It also marked a change in hospital policy. For 75 years, the Annapolis hospital had treated psychiatric patients only on an emergency basis, feeling that they would be better cared for under the purview of the traditional mental hospital system. Now, the short-term, acute care of the mentally ill was seen as a part of the community hospital's responsibility and Anne Arundel General Hospital modified its mission. Eight local psychiatrists chose to become active members of the hospital staff, protocols were written, administrative procedures worked out and in July 1978 the new 12-bed psychiatric unit was opened on the sixth floor of the South Building. The completed sixth floor also housed the special care unit, whose patients were moved from their previous quarters in the 1928 wing (C Building) in April 1978.

The question of a unionized nursing staff arose when, in August 1974, Congress passed an amendment to the Taft-Hartley Labor Act that placed private, not-for-profit voluntary hospitals (like Anne Arundel General Hospital) under the provision of the National Labor Relations Act (NLRA). The local chapter of the Maryland Nurses Association petitioned the National Labor Relations Board (NLRB) for the right to represent Anne Arundel General Hospital nurses. At an election in May 1975, 164 staff nurses voted in favor of the union by a 10-vote majority.

The hospital administration challenged the legality of the election, claiming that the Maryland Nurses Association and its parent organization, the American Nurses Association, included in their membership nurses who were classified as management, thus making these groups ineligible for union status and union protection under the NLRA.

When appeals to the NLRB failed, the hospital's management took its case to the U.S. Court of Appeals in Richmond for what turned out to be a landmark decision. Although Administrator Whittaker admitted to a climate of "minimal hostility" between nurses and management in 1975, he stated that patient care had not suffered. Still, the unresolved matter intensified problems with nurse morale and contract negotiations.

The Appeals Court decision, handed down in 1977, upheld the hospital management's position. It did not solve the basic dispute between the nursing staff and the administration, but it did mean, from the administration's perspective at least, that these problems would be handled from within the hospital's system, without outside pressures.

The issue of the hospital's right to purchase and operate such equipment as it thought necessary for the care and treatment of its patients first surfaced in 1976 when the nuclear medicine department wanted to install a computerized axial tomography (CAT) scanner. Local patients, some seven or eight a week, were being sent to Baltimore for CAT scans; the department's physicians felt that access to this diagnostic marvel should be available in Annapolis. So they bought one. Drs. Barry Friedman, Peter Schilder and Nicholas Capozzoli formed a corporation and contracted with the hospital to lease space for their machine's installation and operation. At the end of five years, they would give it to the hospital.

Approval for the purchase of such expensive machinery was required by the Central Maryland Health Systems Agency, an advisory board to the Maryland Comprehensive Health Planning Agency, which was charged by the state with making sure that hospitals did not overextend themselves financially and push up the cost of medical care. The Anne Arundel General Hospital management figured that there would be no problem with approval since the hospital's growing service population numbered more than 100,000 people and its geographic position and fully qualified specialists made it a reasonable location for a CAT scanner. Besides, the machine was privately owned and operated at no cost to the hospital. They were wrong. State planners did not approve the request for a CAT scanner and in February 1977 the Maryland Health Department threatened to revoke the hospital's license unless the scanner was removed. Thus began another process of appeals through the system. Finally in October 1978, the Maryland Health Department Board of Review ruled in favor of the hospital. The machine could stay.

Fortunately for Anne Arundel General Hospital patients, CAT scans continued during the appeals process. By the time of official approval, the machine had more than justified its value to the hospital's service population.

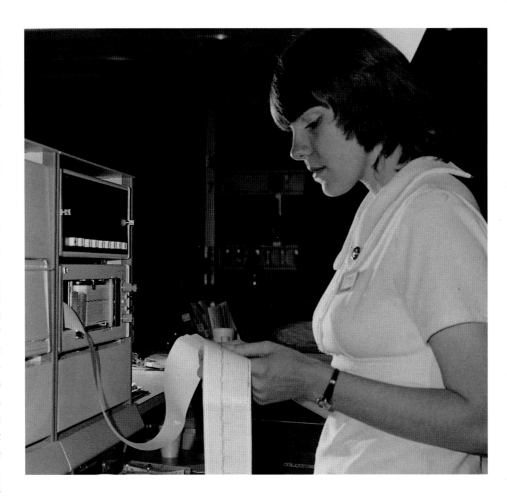

The most intense and emotional controversy the hospital faced in the late 1970s was the parking garage issue. For literally years, the matter was played out in packed meeting rooms, tense board rooms, the pages of local and Baltimore newspapers, on street corners, in private homes—anywhere that Annapolitans got together. Angry words were spoken, feelings were hurt, loyalties pulled this way and that.

Parking in Annapolis goes right to the visceral core of any local resident or driver. It is an unending game of musical parking spaces—without the music and with absolutely no laughter. Parking in Annapolis is serious busi-

New monitoring equipment, like this electrocardiograph read by Lynn Wagner, kept the coronary care unit up to date.

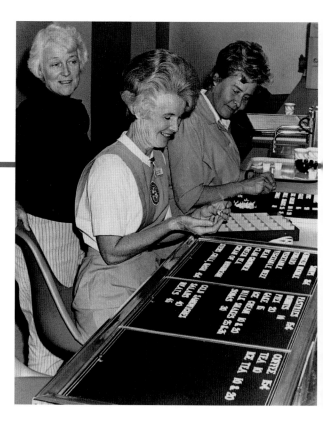

Mrs. Roman Hales (left) and Mrs. Paul Fleishmann, members of the Auxilary, assemble the menu for the new Snack Bar. Mrs. Everett McCleery stands behind. A close inspection of the menu reveals that a cup of coffee cost 15 cents and a small scoop of ice cream cost 10 cents!

ness and in the days before designated parking districts, with their two-hour limit and residential permits, the situation was even worse.

From the hospital's point of view, the proposed parking garage was essential. Permits for the new Cathedral Street wing and the use of the South Building's two extra floors were predicated upon the hospital's providing a specific number of off-street parking spaces. The constant complaints from 1,000 employees, volunteers and physicians, echoed by the often frantic pleas from relatives and friends of patients, made adequate parking facilities critical.

On the other hand, the city's status as a tourist-attracting historic landmark, with all the economic and aesthetic advantages that implied, brought preservation-conscious citizens out in droves to Historic District Commission meetings and planning and zoning hearings. The size and design of the proposed parking garage were topics of heated debate. Residents of the Murray Hill area were divided on the issue; owners with houses overlooking the site tended to oppose the garage, while those who lived on streets coveted by hospital visitors and who had trouble unloading their groceries were more willing to favor it.

Leading the opposition was Historic Annapolis, Inc., under its president, St. Clair Wright. The group's vice president was Pringle Symonds, who also held the chair of the HDC, which consistently rejected the garage plans.

With no compromise possible, the dispute ended up in the courts but continued to be waged in the newspapers throughout 1977 and early 1978. On March 7, 1978, Kent County Judge George B. Raisin, Jr., sitting in

the Anne Arundel County Circuit Court, ruled the HDC denial "arbitrary and capricious." Historic Annapolis filed an appeal; the hospital pursued legislation to exempt its property from the historic district. Finally, after a series of meetings among representatives of the hospital, Historic Annapolis, the city and the Anne Arundel County delegation to the General Assembly, a historic agreement was signed on April 17, 1978, marking the end of the controversy. The hospital could build its garage and would not challenge the historic district boundaries; Historic Annapolis would drop its appeal; and the city officials would back an ordinance limiting the height and bulk of future buildings within the Historic District.

The new five-level, 367-car parking garage on Shaw and South streets opened in September 1979. Hospital personnel thought their parking problems were solved. The building also provided room for a larger Clothes Box showroom, with storage and work rooms and a convenient drop-off area in the garage.

Throughout the 1970s, the Auxiliary maintained most of its traditional services to the hospital and added new ones. Two men, George Schaun and Capt. Donald McClench, joined the Auxiliary in 1969 and

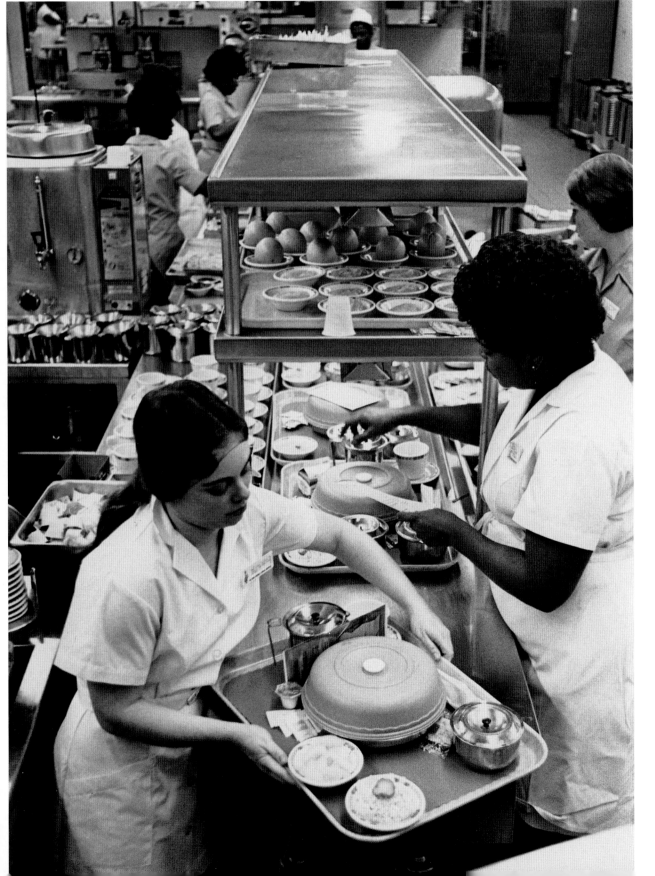

Michal Denowitz, Loretta Pergason and Paula E. Rogers preparing patient trays, 1973.

113

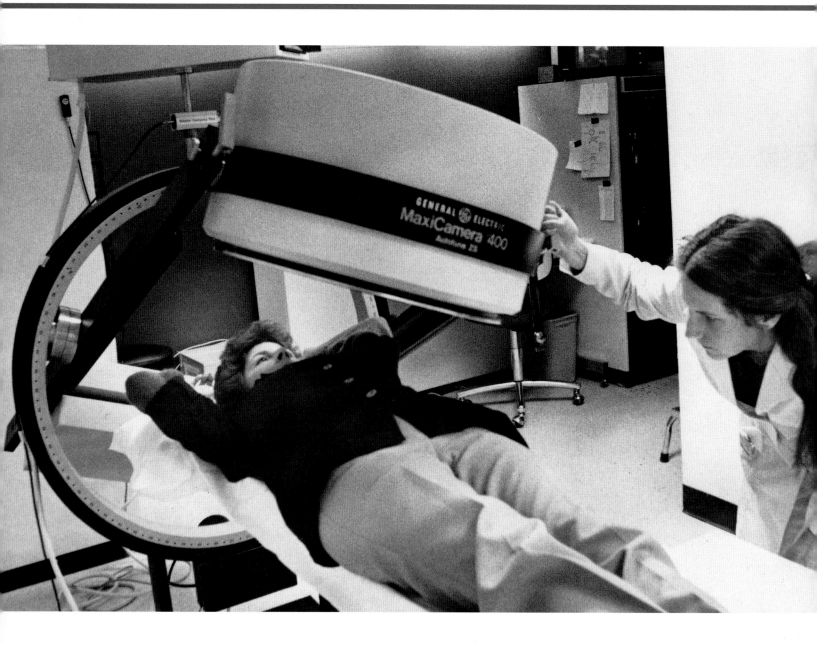

A gamma camera used for scanning in the nuclear medicine department.

immediately added their skills to the hospital's in-house television channel. Mr. Schaun and his wife, Virginia, also an Auxiliary member, began a history project for both the Auxiliary and the hospital in general. They and their committee interviewed former and present members of the medical staff and volunteers and collected newspaper clippings. Informal histories were written in 1971. In

1972, the Auxiliary modified the wording of its bylaws to give its male members, then nine out of a total membership of 916, equal status. While hospital auxiliaries in other areas found it necessary to hire a manager to coordinate volunteer services, the Anne Arundel General Hospital group continued to rely on its own volunteer placement committee to direct the services of the members.

Sponsorship of symphony concerts ended with the 1973–1974 season largely because, with Annapolis's own fine symphony orchestra, there was no longer a need to bring in orchestras from Baltimore or Washington. The days at Laurel Raceway with their popular fashion shows continued to draw crowds and in the fall of 1976 Auxiliary members presented the Holiday Show and Sale, featuring handmade "Auxiliary Originals" and other specialty gifts. In 1976, the Auxiliary made the final payment on its $500,000 pledge to the hospital's building fund, bringing its total building fund contributions to more than $1 million since 1964.

Never content to rest on its laurels, the Auxiliary promptly pledged another $600,000 to the hospital's expansion fund and paid it off completely within two years. These pledges were in addition to the group's annual gifts toward the hospital's operating expenses and to the nursing school and library.

By the end of the decade, the Auxiliary's 1,000 or so members were giving more than 70,000 volunteer hours per year to the hospital.

For all its problems with outside agencies, Anne Arundel General Hospital continued through the 1970s to attract physicians trained and experienced in a variety of specialties and subspecialties: oncology, neurology, neurosurgery, vascular and chest surgery, hematology, nephrology, endocrinology. In 1977, with 146 active staff physicians and 30 on the courtesy staff, there was talk of closing the staff in some services.

The hospital also continued to increase its patient load, with more than 11,500 admissions to the 240 beds in 1976 and more than 12,000 admissions to 269 beds in 1979. Emergency patients increased from 33,739 to 34,526 and hospital births rose from 1,376 to 1,789 over the same three-year period. The average stay in the hospital was about six days.

Revenues from all services in 1976–1979 generally outpaced expenses by 2-5 percent. The hospital's annual budget topped $17 million in 1979.

At the annual meeting of the Annapolis Emergency Hospital Association in March 1978, members approved a bylaw changing the association's name to the Anne Arundel General Hospital, Inc. The official amendment to the corporation papers was made on April 25, 1978. This was the first of several corporate changes that would be made over the years ahead. Also at that time, a bylaw moving the annual meeting to September was adopted.

Eighteen months later, at the next association meeting in September 1979, members heard the last report of their long-time administrator, Lyman C. Whittaker. After 22 years, "Whit" was retiring. This hardworking, imaginative, ever-enthusiastic man, who had led the hospital through its crucial years of change, left the association and the board with a challenge for the future:

"While we are leaders in hospital facilities, programs, health care and finances, we lag seriously behind in our outdated and antiquated corporate structure. It should and must keep moving towards an updated structure so the board's efforts are able to respond adequately to today's complex needs."

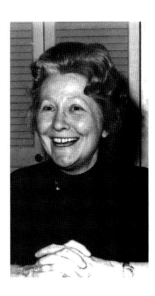

Rebecca M. Clatanoff, **Auxiliary volunteer and member of the hospital's Board of Managers.**

Anne Arundel Medical Center has been a family affair for the Achenbacks.

I worked there for 45 years, and all three of my daughters have worked there at some point; two still do. I came to Annapolis after I graduated from nursing school in Baltimore; I wanted to be an OR nurse but they didn't have an opening there, so they put me with the kids and that's where I stayed.

The hospital was pretty primitive at first; we were sterilizing things in fish kettles. Visiting hours for the children's ward was for two hours on Sundays and Wednesdays—that was it! No parents stayed overnight. But we had enough nurses to do one-on-one care, and the doctors stayed right there with the really sick kids. It was a fun time; everyone helped and there was teamwork right down to the bone. There were some excellent doctors and nurses.

When the new building opened in 1970, it was a whole new day. We had so much room that we thought we'd walk ourselves to death. Around that time the nursing hats went, we started wearing colored tops and white pants, and started wearing tennis shoes.

The biggest difference was that the parents were allowed to stay, because there were all private rooms. It was better for the kids, and it helped the nurses, too. Now we encourage parents to stay so the child feels more secure.

The nurses came into their own towards the end of the 1980s. The Nursing Council came into play, and I even sat on the Board of Directors for the hospital. A lot of new doctors were coming in, and members of the 'Old Guard' were retiring. Most all of the long-term nurses left then, too. There were a lot of good nurses who laid the groundwork for nursing as it is today at AAMC.

I loved going to work. Now I miss the parents and the kids. Some of my former patients have brought their own kids in to meet me! I still think about many of my patients. I wouldn't want to do anything else but be a nurse. I have lots of happy memories.

Perspective...

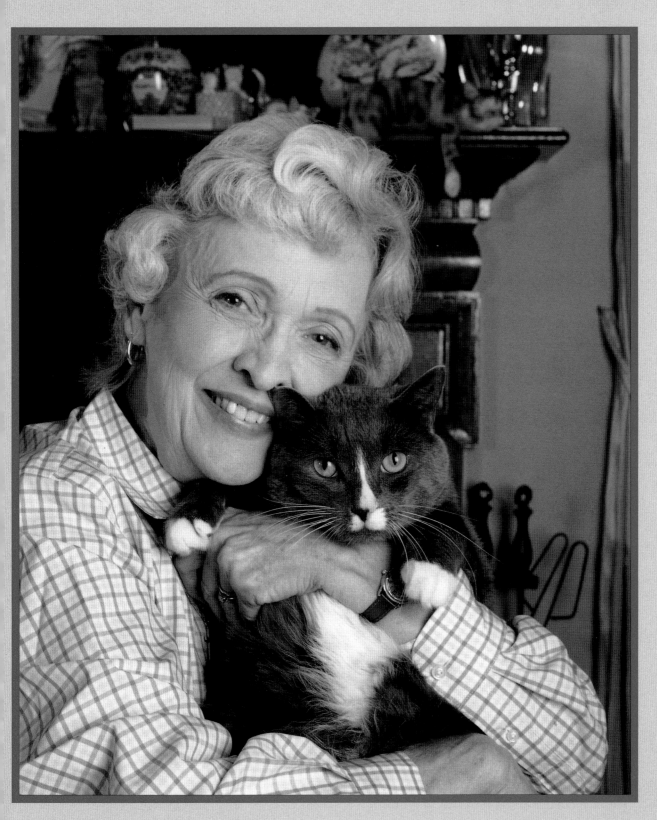

Nancy Achenback, R.N.

Pediatric nurse, 1953-1998

Auxiliary member, 1997-present

Member of AAMC Board of Directors, 1988

Mother of Juli Pastrana, R.N., case manager, Center for Joint Replacement

Mother of Donna Forrester, medical secretary, Center for Joint Replacement

With the opening of the parking garage in 1979 and the last beds of the South, or A, Building in place by 1980, the Anne Arundel General Hospital facility in downtown Annapolis was complete. Any further expansion would have to take place off site. And, given the apparently unceasing spiral of population growth in the county and the increasing sophistication of hospital medicine, expansion would surely be necessary.

For the moment, however, the hospital turned its attention to internal matters. Carl A. Brunetto, assistant administrator since 1959 and known to all as "Chuck," became administrator upon the resignation of Mr. Whittaker. Martin L. "Chip" Doordan stepped up as his assistant. Mr. Doordan had come to the hospital in 1972 as a graduate student in health care administration at George Washington University and had remained after completing his master's degree. At a time when most hospitals saw an almost yearly turnover in their administrative officers, Anne Arundel General Hospital had the advantage of a well-liked, well-trained junior staff ready to take the reins. In the words of Carl Brunetto:

"I think it's a compliment to the hospital and to the board and to the community, because it takes all those people to keep someone here [that long]. . . There are not any dramatic changes. Basically our programs continue to move forward. . . and I think that's why this organization has been so successful. And we are successful, there isn't any question about that, and we provide just excellent, excellent care."

Even the most genial and experienced administrator could not completely diffuse tensions between the medical staff and the Board of Managers in the early 1980s. Central to the dispute was the board's decision in 1980 to combine the departments of radiology and nuclear medicine into a new department of imaging. When the new chief was unable to reach contract agreements with five staff radiologists, they were forced to leave the hospital and were replaced by new staff. Suits were filed by three of the original radiologists, two left the area and angry words were spoken on both sides.

The medical staff felt it had not been appropriately apprised of the board's plans. The board upheld its privilege to create departments within the hospital. Both agreed on the need for better communications. Damage had been done, not only to individuals, but also to the department that offered such promise in the use of medical science's most exciting new diagnostic equipment. Over the next year, radiology referrals to the hospital dropped dramatically as several private outpatient radiology offices opened in the Annapolis area. The potential of reduced radiology facilities for hospital inpatients coupled with the marked decrease in hospital income from the department were of concern to both the medical staff and the board. After two years of meetings and planning, a new, reorganized department of radiological services, to include radiology, ultrasonography, nuclear medicine and computerized scanning, was created under a new chief of service. Two of the radiologists who had left in 1980 returned to the hospital staff.

Another result of the radiology dispute was a change in the composition of the Board of Managers. Not only were new faces brought in from the community, but by 1982, the pres-

THE MEDICAL CENTER
1980 - 1991

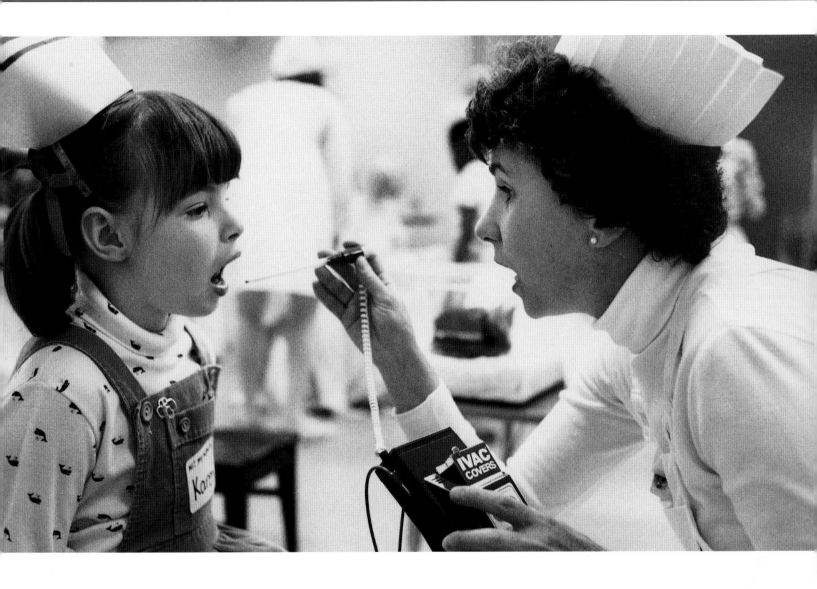

ident of the medical staff became an *ex officio* board member.

Long-range planning occupied hospital management and staff through much of 1981. Anne Arundel General Hospital was determined to keep abreast of developments in medical science and community needs and ahead of the demand for services. Several factors influenced plans: the increasingly sophisticated technology for both diagnosis and treatment of medical and psychiatric

problems, the trend toward wellness care and prevention of illnesses, the availability of nursing staff, the limitations of the downtown location and existing physical plant, and the hospital's financial resources. These concerns were not new, but in drawing up what management hoped would be a workable 10-year plan, they had to be reevaluated.

Already affecting hospital admissions were innovative and complex surgical procedures being performed by local physicians. Total

AAMC's Hands on Health program for children was started by pediatric nurse Nancy Achenback in 1979 to familiarize Anne Arundel County kindergarten students with health issues and simple hospital procedures.

An aerial view of the downtown campus of Anne Arundel General Hospital, c.1985.

hip or knee replacement, percutaneous kidney stone surgery and revascularization procedures promised a longer, useful life for elderly, severely ill or traumatized patients. Recent hospital purchases such as a neonatal monitor, operating microscope, bronchoscope, and telemetry and arterial monitors were important aids to physicians and nurses. As technology advanced, other equipment would play an important role in the hospital.

Perhaps the most difficult factors for the hospital to assess in developing a 10-year plan were the changes in the basic philosophy of health care being discussed nationally in the medical and popular press. To some extent, it seemed that the pendulum was swinging back to 19th-century attitudes: illness as a consequence of lifestyle and home-based care preferred for the treatment of the chronically and terminally ill. The nation's concern with

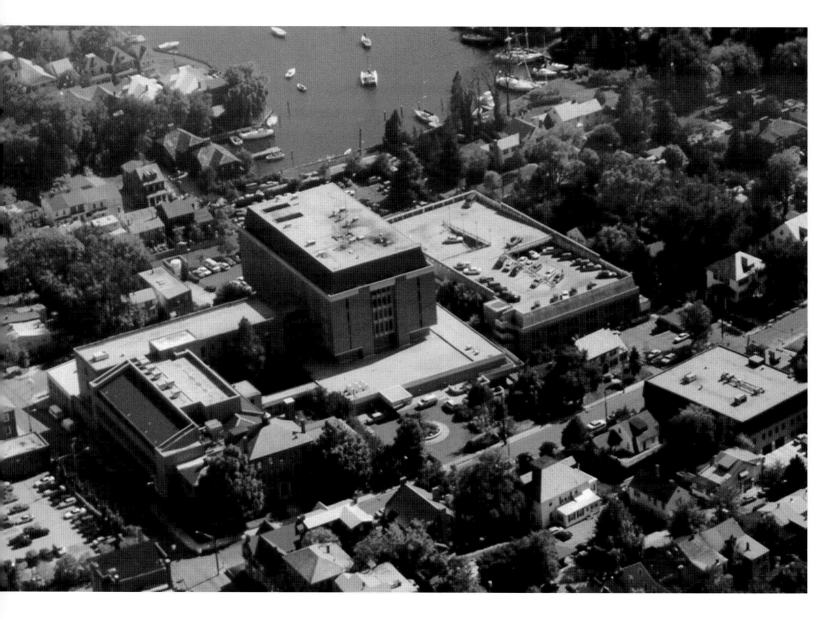

these matters was clear; what was not so clear was the role of the community hospital.

The policy makers of Anne Arundel General Hospital decided that their mission to provide health care to the community did not begin at the hospital's doors, nor did it end there. They believed that hospital sponsorship of educational programs in preventive medicine, health management and home care of the ill was appropriate. Through its in-house television programs and classes for new parents, Anne Arundel General Hospital had been educating the public for several years. Now these efforts would be extended.

In April 1980, the hospital hosted the first Greater Annapolis Health Fair with 20 community health organizations participating and free tests offered for anemia, blood pressure, certain types of cancer and other diseases. The first Healthscope seminars drew interested members of the community to the hospital's new meeting room with topics such as "Hospitals: Where Do All the Dollars Go?" Both programs became annual events, promoting good health as well as good public relations. Hospital physicians and nurses were accustomed to speaking at professional meetings; now a formal speakers bureau made it easier for local organizations to present well-informed programs on health care issues.

In October 1981, Anne Arundel General was given permission by the state to accept a hospice program begun privately by a group of physicians, nurses, clergymen, pastoral counselors and concerned citizens in 1979. Members of the original hospice group became an advisory board to the hospital program, under which 20 physicians and 73 trained volunteers provided care and support to terminally ill patients and their families in

their home environment. For individuals living alone and anxious for emergency assistance in case of falls or sudden illness, the Lifeline program offered immediate contact with the outside world via a battery-operated message sender.

The next years brought the hospital further into the areas of education and support. Several new programs distributed Anne Arundel General Hospital health care information about its services throughout the community. In addition to the pediatric pre-hospitalization program, pediatric nurses instituted hospital visits for kindergarten and preschool classes. Tel-med, a taped telephone information service, opened in 1983 and the D-O-C-S Information Service began in 1987. The hospital encouraged exercise with the Heart Hike measured mile at Annapolis Mall in 1984. To keep public officials abreast of medical developments and the work of the hospital, an annual legislative dinner was inaugurated in 1985.

Outpatient IV medication, initiated in 1983, was a pioneer program used as a model by other institutions and Medicare planners. This and other home-based therapy and support systems, including the home health care program begun in 1984, allowed patients to receive treatment at home, thus reducing the cost of health care to both the patient and the hospital.

In November 1986, the hospital hired its first chaplain and opened the department of pastoral care to provide nondenominational pastoral counseling to patients and their families. The clinical pastoral education program began with five interns in 1988.

Bringing the outside world to the hospital was accomplished with the library's on-line linkage in 1985 to the worldwide data bases of the National Library of Medicine. This on-line service, called MEDLINE, provided easy access to all information pertaining to a particular subject and was of special value in the diagnosis and treatment of unusual diseases or complications. DOCLINE, added in 1986, facilitated interlibrary loans. Funding for the library and its specially trained professional librarian came not only from the hospital budget but also from the medical staff, the Auxiliary and contributions given in memory of deceased physicians.

Deficits in the early 1980s underscored the hospital's continuing need for a secure financial base. In the summer of 1982, the Board of Managers approved the formation of the Anne Arundel General Hospital Foundation, Inc. as an agency to generate and manage voluntary contributions to the hospital, thus separating gifts from operating revenue. The Foundation, incorporated in 1983, would also be charged with raising the millions of dollars necessary for the hospital to carry out its long-range plans.

Not that all the hospital's contributions were money. As it had for so many years, the community still brought patients those little treats that made an institutional stay more personal. Valentine's Day tray favors handmade by Brownie troops and Belvedere School second graders and the First Baptist Church in 1981, for instance, or the visits by clowns, choral groups and Girl Scouts brightened a patient's day.

As nursing administration diversified and floor registered nurses became an endangered species in many parts of the nation during the late 1970s, Anne Arundel General felt itself fortunate that it did not have a serious shortage of qualified

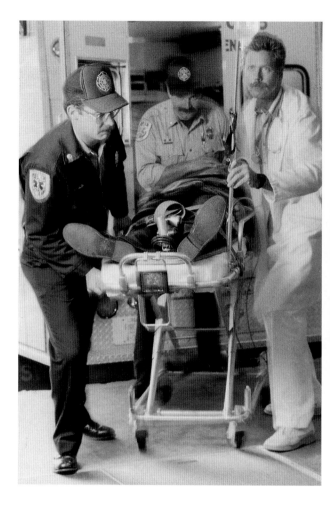

nurses. By the early 1980s, however, the hospital was hard pressed to find and keep good nurses.

Primary nursing, implemented in three areas in 1981, had a positive effect on morale. Assigned registered nurses took on the full responsibility of planning the nursing care for specific patients, working closely with the physician, dietitian and other health care providers, as well as the patient and the patient's family. Other members of the patient's nursing team followed the care plan of the primary nurse. The opportunity for continuity of care and increased accountability appealed to many nurses who often felt themselves somewhat removed from close patient contact.

While the representatives of the board, the administration and the medical staff pondered an extension of the hospital's facilities off site, changes were made to streamline and improve the operation of the downtown buildings. In 1983, biomedical safety, security and maintenance were grouped into a new engineering department. Also that year, two rooms in the X-ray area were renovated and equipped at a cost of $1.6 million and a new CAT scanner was purchased for another $1.4 million. A new fire alarm system and renovations in the lab and lobby were part of the continuing improvements to the physical plant. The landscaping committee of the Auxiliary brought gardening talents to bear on the grounds of the main entrance.

In 1984, the hospital began the implementation of its long-range plans with the purchase for $3 million of 104 acres on Jennifer Road near Route 50 and the Annapolis Mall. This site would provide space to expand the hospital's services beyond the confines of the downtown site. Some people said that the board should have taken this step 20 years earlier when the subject first came up; others feared that dividing the hospital's services would add pressure to the medical staff and the burden of duplicated services to the hospital's finances. The board believed, however, that the cost was advantageous and the expansion inevitable.

During the same period, the hospital's managers authorized the purchase of two privately owned radiology offices for convenient outpatient access. These facilities, one on Riva Road and one on Ritchie Highway in Arnold, were taken over by the hospital in

1985, and in September of that year a breast cancer diagnostic clinic was set up in the Arnold office. Planned were three additional walk-in clinics—in Crofton, Severna Park and on Kent Island—to offer outpatient care under the broadening wing of the hospital.

This satellite center concept was part of the 10-year plan advised by the hospital planning firm of Herman Smith Associates to which the Board of Managers had turned for specific advice on reaching its long-term goals. The continued life of the hospital would depend upon its ability to meet the challenges, or threats, of what was seen by many as a revolution in this nation's health care system. By the mid-1980s, cost containment regulations of federal and state agencies and private insurers had drastically reduced hospital occupancy rates. Medical procedures that a few years before would have necessitated a

Donald M. Klein, a physician's assistant in the emergency department, comforts a young patient, 1992.

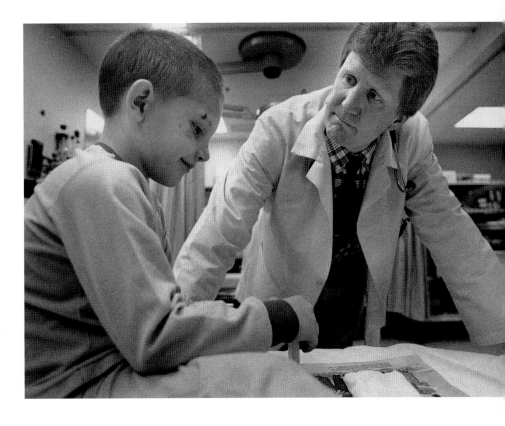

For the community, establishing an oncology program and developing a large, well-trained, research-oriented team to treat malignancy in Annapolis has been an accomplishment.

Dr. Stanley P. Watkins, Jr
November 26, 1991

hospital stay of several days were now being done on an outpatient basis. Hospitals were thrown into direct competition with health maintenance organizations, private walk-in clinics and the satellite centers of neighboring hospitals.

In some parts of Maryland, hospitals were in serious financial trouble, forced to maintain a large multiservice facility in the face of shrinking admissions. Because of its location in the midst of a still-growing area and because of its reputation for high-level health care, Anne Arundel General Hospital was one of only

Roscoe Davis in the laboratory, 1982.

Computers help Dr. Cornelia M. Dettmer, radiation oncology specialist; and Robert Siddon, Ph.D., physicist, review oncology cases.

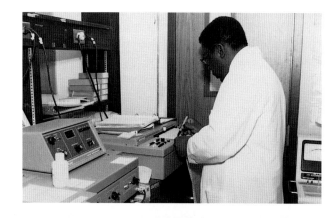

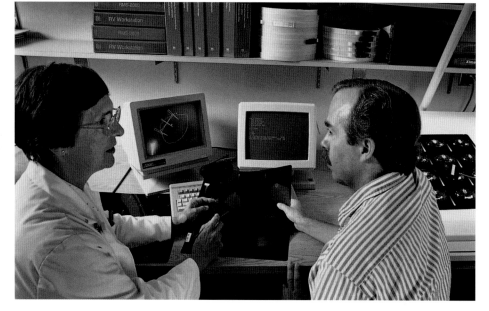

three Maryland hospitals with increased admissions in 1984. Nevertheless, with the county's growth rate slowing to about 13 percent in the 1980s, compared with the 20–30 percent growth of the previous two decades, hospital officers were concerned. Caught between the requirements of outside regulatory agencies and their own determination to provide good, modern medical care, the hospital and its physicians found themselves thoroughly mired in the national health care crisis. Increased provisions for outpatient diagnosis and treatment seemed a reasonable solution to the immediate problem.

Justification for both this concern and the emphasis on outpatient facilities came in 1985 when, for probably the first time in the history of the Annapolis hospital, patient admissions dropped by roughly 2 percent. In sharp contrast, use of the outpatient diagnostic and surgical facilities increased that year by an overall average of 37 percent.

The hospital's medical staff changed in both composition and membership during the mid-1980s. Podiatry was established as a service in 1985 and family practice split off from the medical service in 1984.

Staff committees—quality assurance, utilization review, infections, tumor and others—continued to devote hours of time to making sure that the medical staff not only delivered top-quality care but did so at the lowest possible cost. A special staff committee on AIDS was formed in 1987 to initiate protective policies for hospital personnel and to ensure proper care for AIDS patients.

By 1987, the hospital had 274 medical staff members and the credentials committee was receiving applications regularly. A number of

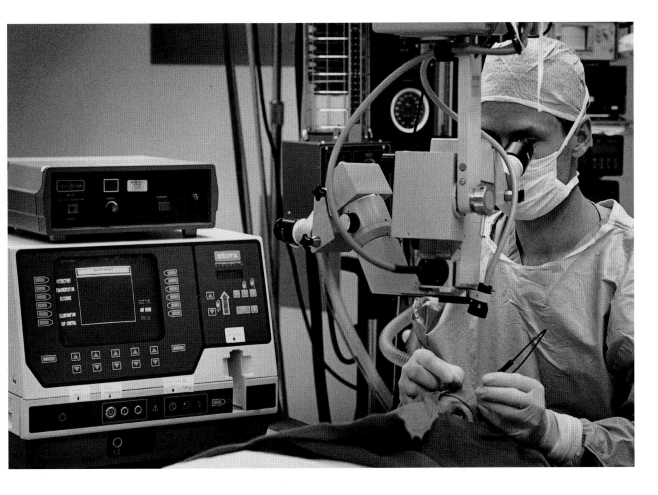

the senior doctors on the staff—men and women who had practiced in the hospital since the 1940s or 1950s and had seen it and medical science change so dramatically over the years—retired from active practice in the mid-1980s. The crisis in malpractice insurance caused two ob/gyn specialists to give up their practices entirely and five others to drop their obstetrics privileges. This left only 15 obstetricians on the staff to deliver the 2,000 or so babies born annually in the hospital.

Complicating the problem in countywide obstetrical care was the county health department's loss of obstetricians for its clinics. For some years, Johns Hopkins Hospital had pro-

vided obstetrical services to the 400–450 expectant mothers using county clinics in Anne Arundel General's service area. In 1987, however, Hopkins indicated that it would no longer serve these maternity clinics. Anne Arundel County and Anne Arundel General Hospital officials worked out a plan to attract more local obstetricians and to allow Anne Arundel General Hospital to give the full range of prenatal, delivery and postnatal care required for these patients. In 1987–1988, almost 300 babies were born in the Annapolis hospital under this program. Unfortunately, many of them were high-risk babies, born to mothers whose age, poor health or use of drugs created problems for their infants.

NO ONE INDIVIDUAL COULD EVER RECEIVE OR RIGHTLY DESERVE CREDIT FOR ANY MAJOR, SIGNIFICANT PROGRAM. IT IS REALLY A TEAM EFFORT OF MANY, MANY TALENTS: THE DOCTORS, THE ADMINISTRATIVE STAFF, THE EMPLOYEES, THE BOARD, THE VOLUNTEERS. AND THAT TRULY IS THE SUCCESS OF OUR HOSPITAL.

CARL A. BRUNETTO, PRESIDENT, AAGHCS
November 21, 1991

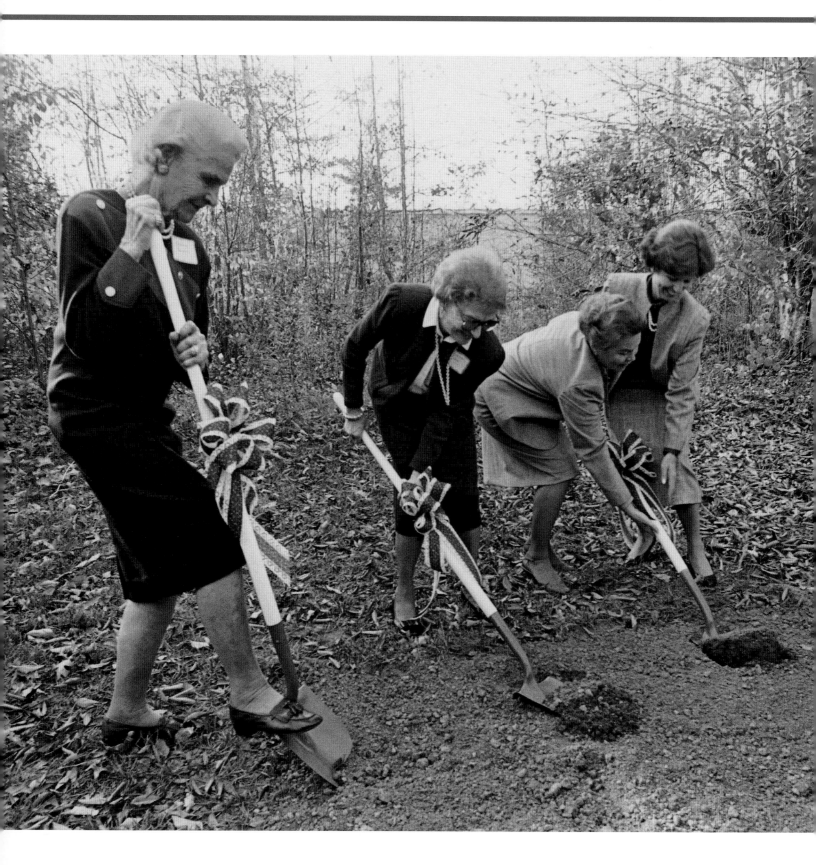

Because of the greater number of newborns requiring immediate care and because, in general, children admitted to the hospital were more likely to be seriously ill, staff pediatricians felt that the presence of a full-time pediatrician was warranted. Two local pediatricians contracted with the hospital to provide the coverage and the program began in December 1987 with four fully qualified pediatric specialists.

The first use of the Jennifer Road land was as the site of the hospital's magnetic resonance imager (MRI), the first hospital-based MRI in the state, which began screening patients in 1986. Architects RTKL drew up plans in 1986 and 1987 for oncology and outpatient surgical centers, the first buildings of the new outpatient treatment complex.

Since the hospital did not plan to use the entire 104 acres of land, the board sold 19 acres to the State Highway Commission for $5.2 million so that a convenient interchange could be built connecting Jennifer Road and the mall with the redesigned Route 50. The 34 acres remaining on the south side of Jennifer Road would be considered part of the county's Parole Town Center, and Rouse and Associates was hired in 1989 to develop the property. Income from the development was designated to secure the hospital's financial base and fund further capital improvement projects on the hospital's 52 acres to the north of Jennifer Road.

A massive fundraising drive by the Foundation and the board to finance construction of the oncology and ambulatory surgery centers and a health education center on Jennifer Road soon reached its $6 million goal. Of special concern to the hospital and the community was the availability of cancer treatments close to home—not just in Baltimore and Washington as was then the case. Individuals, civic organizations and county businesses contributed generously for the new facility.

With such public support, the hospital arranged a bond issue to gather the additional money to begin the $13 million project. With Gardiner and Gardiner as construction manager, ground for the first building was broken in November 1987.

By 1988, Anne Arundel General Hospital was not just the familiar complex of buildings on Franklin Street. It was also full-service outpatient radiology offices on

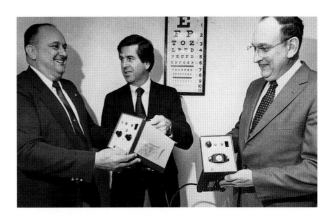

Caroline Baldwin, Elizabeth Mitchell, Margaret Ellis and Ruby Fuller dig in at the ground-breaking ceremonies for Medical Park, November 8, 1987 (opposite).

Lions Club of Annapolis members Charles Steele (left) and Richard Achenbach (right) present Martin L. Doordan, hospital associate administrator with a gift of ophthalmological equipment, 1983.

Proceeds of the 1983 "Big Raffle" are given to hospital administrator Carl A. Brunetto in the form of a large check by co-chairmen Donna Olfson, Rebecca Clatanoff and Mary Hiltabidle.

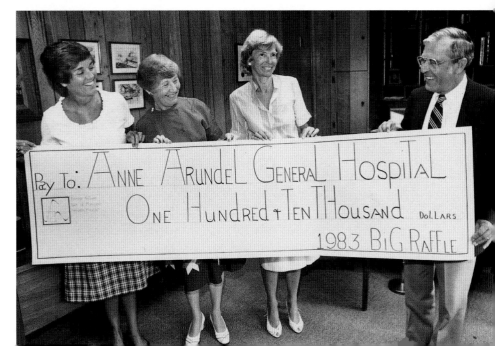

Riva Road and Ritchie Highway, at Crofton, and, in December, on Kent Island—all four operating under the name Anne Arundel Diagnostics. It was also three outpatient centers, in Severna Park, Crofton and on Kent Island, called Anne Arundel Walk-in Health Centers and opened in 1987 and 1988. And, in just one year, it would also be the new treatment and education centers on Jennifer Road to be called Medical Park.

The detailed management and supervision required by what had grown into a very complex operation could not be carried by one Board of Managers—or one administrative staff. It was time for a restructuring of the corporation and some new names.

Just as the hospital's name had changed in 1949 from Annapolis Emergency Hospital to Anne Arundel General Hospital to reflect changes in its service and community, so the name changed again in March 1988 to Anne Arundel General Hospital and Medical Center.

The modern institution was both a hospital and the complex of ancillary departments that constitute a regional medical center. At the same time, the volunteer Board of Managers became, instead, the Board of Trustees of a parent corporation: Anne Arundel General Health Care Systems, Inc., reflecting again the changes in their duties and responsibilities. Not for many years had board members checked for dust on hospital windowsills or ordered canned goods for the kitchen and coal for the furnaces. The board now functioned as policy makers and long-range planners—that is, as trustees—and it was appropriate for them to be named so. The hospital would continue to have its own Board of Directors chosen from the Board of Trustees.

Under the aegis of the parent corporation, then, came the newly renamed hospital, including the facilities at Medical Park, the fundraising Foundation, a management company responsible for the development of the nonmedical part of the Jennifer Road property, and service companies to manage the diagnostic and walk-in centers. The system was designed to be responsive to additional changes in the health care environment.

The new corporate structure necessitated changes in administrative personnel. On August 1, 1988, Carl A. Brunetto became president and chief executive officer of Anne Arundel General Health Care Systems, Inc., with overall responsibilities for the entire organization and Martin L. Doordan assumed the position of president and chief executive officer of the Anne Arundel General Hospital and Medical Center. The hospital's new name proved to be too cumbersome for comfort and within a year it was shortened to Anne Arundel Medical Center.

During all of the corporate reorganization of the late 1980s, the hospital, under its various names, remained a hospital—caring for more than 14,000 inpatients a year in its 303-bed Franklin Street facility and treating another 36,000 in its emergency room. Laboratory procedures passed the one million mark annually and more than 2,500 babies were born in the hospital in 1988.

After 30 years of continuous accreditation by the Joint Commission on the Accreditation of Hospitals and its successor, the Joint Commission on the Accreditation of Healthcare Organizations, Anne Arundel General Hospital received word in May 1988 that its "deemed" status was being revoked—not by the Joint Commission, but by the Health Care

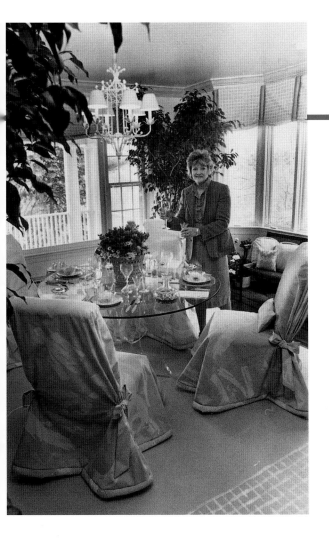

The HCFA decision regarding Anne Arundel General was based on reports from the Department of Licensing and Certification of the state health department. Prompted by two complaints, a state inspection of the hospital in March 1988 found deficiencies in the documentation of emergency room quality assurance. Quality assurance meant, basically, the medical staff's systematic and continuing review of cases to determine that appropriate diagnosis and treatment had taken place and that, if a problem were found, procedures were implemented to make sure it did not happen again. Federal authorities notified the press and then the hospital that its deemed status had been withdrawn. The general public responded immediately with letters to *The Capital* defending the hospital, but several similar complaints were received. The hospital staff continued its efforts to correct the documentation problem and appealed the HCFA ruling.

In late May, HCFA sent a team of 13 state and federal inspectors to Annapolis. For two-and-a-half days, they investigated all aspects of the hospital from fire safety to nursing and physician care and reviewed the required documentation for each case questioned. Their findings resulted in an announcement on June 7 that Anne Arundel General Hospital was in full compliance with all the 20 conditions of participation in the Medicare program and that the hospital's deemed status would be restored. That the hospital was able to satisfy the federal and state requirements in only one month underscored the fact that only its documentation had been at issue, not the quality of actual patient care. At no time had the hospital lost its Joint Commission accreditation or its privilege to admit and treat Medicare patients.

The national nursing shortage in the late

Financing Administration (HCFA) of the federal government. HCFA, an agency under the Department of Health and Human Services, administered the Medicare program and the federal government's participation in Medicaid. Customarily, a hospital fully accredited by the Joint Commission was automatically "deemed" to meet HCFA standards as a provider of hospital services to Medicare patients.

However, under certain circumstances, HCFA could revoke the deemed status and place a hospital under the supervision of the state health department, which would make regular inspections until the deficiencies were corrected or, if not corrected, until the hospital was declared ineligible for Medicare participation. The correction period might last three months to a year. Loss of the deemed status was a serious matter.

Delica Mathews and friend, 1980. In 1976, Delica was the first baby born in the hospital's new maternity wing.

The Hemminger quadruplets, born on October 9, 1980, return to Anne Arundel General Hospital to celebrate their first birthday. From left: Andrew, Mrs. Hemminger, Beverly, Beth, Daniel, Mr. Hemminger and Christine. Older sister Michelle is in front.

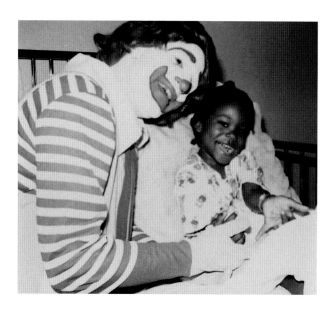

1980s continued to concern physicians, supervisors and administrators. In 1989, Anne Arundel Medical Center became one of the first institutions in the country to form a professional nursing council. Nurse representatives on the council would participate in meetings of the joint conference committee and the Board of Directors when nursing issues were under discussion. A formal collaborative practice committee brought nurses and doctors together to plan for improvements in patient care.

Hospital employees numbered more than 1,600 in 1989 and there were times when some felt underpaid and discriminated against. A child care referral service, new merit program and a renovated employee lounge addressed complaints, and sponsorship of an adult education program broadened career options for employees. Developmentally disabled clients of the Providence Center and students of the Central Special School were given the opportunity to work in the hospital and gain valuable experience.

The hospital was a major regional business, with operating expenses of more than $56 million a year in 1989. But the hospital's business was still people—people in trouble, in pain, people with medical needs—and the staff cared for them.

Always, too, there were the pink-clad ladies and gentlemen of the Auxiliary helping out, taking care of extras, smiling behind the snack bar counter, raising money. The 1,000 or so Auxiliary members gave more than 76,000 hours of time to the hospital in 1986 and 1,000 hours more than that in 1988. Junior volunteers still came to the hospital each year to see what nursing was all about. A number of them found that this was the career they wanted.

The Auxiliary's fundraising events included a semi-annual Designer Show House, begun in 1980, as well as the Pink Lady Ball, Clothes Box, fashion shows and the winter Tree of Lights, which illuminated the hospital's grounds at the holiday season. In 1987, the Auxiliary took over the Big Raffle in its fourth year as a major hospital fundraiser. The following year, the Auxiliary installed a flower-vending machine in the lobby. Auxiliary pledges to the hospital and Medical Park for the 1980s totaled $2.75 million. By May of 1992, the Auxiliary had given over $6 million to the hospital during its 48 years of existence.

The downtown hospital was not forgotten during the construction off site. Renovations to the emergency service area, new birthing rooms in the labor and delivery suite and improvements in the physical therapy department were all accomplished in 1989. In 1990, the hospice unit within the hospital, first financed by Mrs. J. Walter Jones in 1986 in memory of her late husband, was increased to

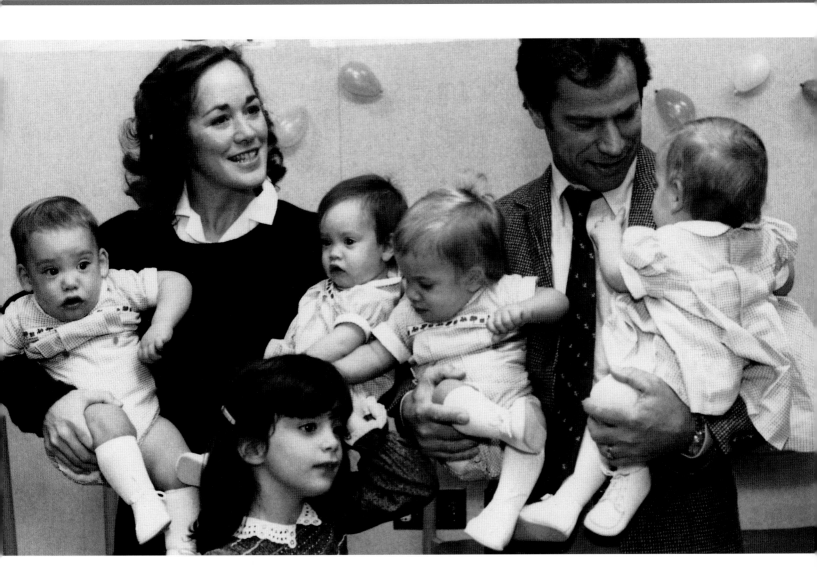

four rooms. Environmental concerns led to an energy management system, funded by the U.S. Department of Energy, and the use of a retort sterilizer to shred needles and prepare medical waste for safe disposal. As various services relocated to Medical Park in the 1990s, further renovations and additions would be made to the downtown facility.

On October 15, 1989, Medical Park dedicated its oncology and outpatient surgery centers and the health education building. The com-

puterized scanning procedures and treatments in the new oncology center offered local cancer patients state-of-the-art care close to home. The surgical facility included four modern operating suites, recovery rooms and a comfortable waiting room. Completion of the health education center provided space for more than 50 different types of classes ranging from aerobics to stress relief, CPR, child care and health management.

Anne Arundel Diagnostics centers in Crofton,

Arnold and Annapolis continued to provide outpatient radiology services in easily accessible locations, but the Kent Island radiology center and all of the walk-in centers were closed in 1990 and 1991 because they had become financially impractical. Another casualty of the recessive economy of the early 1990s was development of the commercial area across Jennifer Road from Medical Park. Due to the economic climate in 1991, Rouse and Associates decided not to carry through its commitment to this project and the relationship was terminated. The hospital's Board of Trustees decided to wait for a more stable economy before proceeding with any future plans for the land.

In addition to Medical Park and the diagnostic centers, Anne Arundel General Health Care Systems joined with the county and state to offer treatment to teens and young adults suffering from substance abuse. The growing numbers of Anne Arundel County young people with drug and alcohol problems and the lack of nearby residential treatment centers made it imperative for government officials to concern themselves with this issue. In 1990, the county donated eight acres of land on Riva Road and $2 million, and the state added $2.5 million for a new facility to be called Pathways. It would be administered and staffed by AAMC, thus confirming the hospital's dedication to the medical needs of the community.

Changes in the structure of the Board of Trustees for Anne Arundel General Health Care Systems were approved at the annual meeting in September 1991. Under the amended bylaws, the committee on trusteeship would receive nominations and recommend to the board for election those individuals whose particular talents, skills and experience would best serve the needs of the

organization. The board would then elect its own new members. The number of trustees was increased from 15 to 16, with four members elected each year for four-year terms. After two continuous terms, a trustee would have to remain off the board for two years before serving only one additional term, thus limiting the total board service for any one individual to 12 years. The new bylaws also provided for additional *ex officio* members: the president of Anne Arundel Medical Center and another representative of the medical staff.

As the hospital entered its 90th year of operation in the summer of 1991, the original ladies of the board would never have recognized the institution they founded at the beginning of the century. Their simple cottage hospital had become a multimillion-dollar complex. The 39,601 patients who used the Franklin Street emergency services during 1990–91 were just 19 people short of the entire county's population in 1900. The 15,965 inpatients and 2,917 births that year would have been incomprehensible even in a major municipal hospital in 1902. And it was far more than a mere hospital—it was a true health system with satellite outpatient centers, extensive community outreach and a growing presence at Medical Park.

"Everyone was reminded that a decision will have to be made as to what development will take place at Medical Park and what renovations will be made to the downtown facility."

AAGHCS Board of Trustees
February 1991 meeting minutes

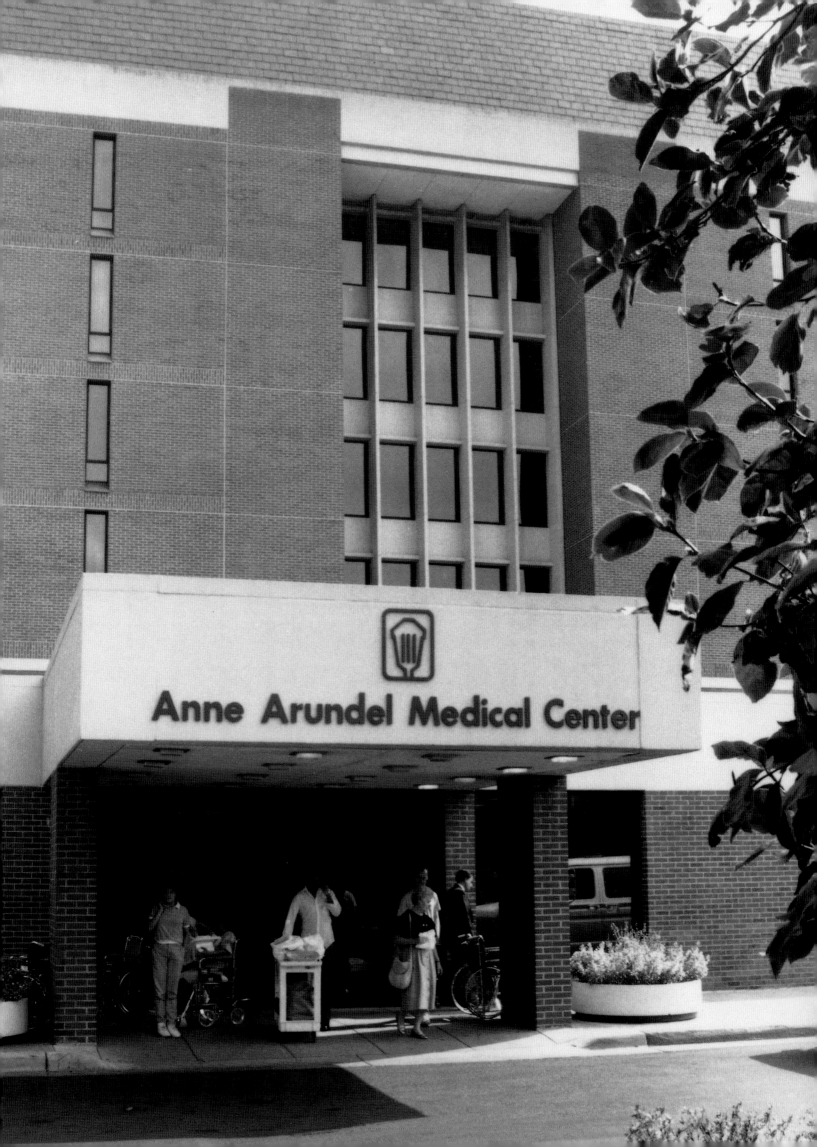

I grew up in Annapolis on Conduit Street. My great uncle, Dr. Walton Hopkins, was one of the first physicians on the medical staff.

My mother was in the Auxiliary and was co-chair of the first Pink Lady Ball. I had my tonsils out at the hospital in 1950, and my two younger children were born here. So the hospital always has been a part of my life.

When I first was elected to the board in 1985, it was still the Board of Managers. We were involved in all aspects of the day-to-day business of the hospital. In the late 1980s, the philosophy changed. We became more educated about the best way to fulfill our obligations, so we became a Board of Trustees to manage the governance of the hospital. We try to get a good balance of individuals on the board, with diversity of expertise and racial and ethnic diversity, too. We look for people with different perspectives, a desire to serve and the ability to devote time.

It took a very professional board to make the decisions we had to make in the 1990s. We developed the Clatanoff and Wayson Pavilions and then we decided to build a new hospital. We looked into the possibility of networking with other hospitals, but ultimately decided against merging. We also approved the allocation of resources for many important clinical initiatives.

A hospital is like a three-legged stool—it takes the medical staff, the administration and the board to work properly. One party gets an idea and the other two legs help decide if it's in the best interests of the community. Over the years, we've become more and more efficient in working together. Sometimes there's a lot of discussion about a particular issue, but people always agree when it comes down to the mission of the hospital and community health.

I'm struck by the unselfishness of board members in doing what's best for the community. In my time on the board, I've learned a lot about the health care industry and I've met a lot of truly great people. I'd have to say my proudest moment as board chairman was when I got to announce that we were naming the Women's and Children's Pavilion for Becky Clatanoff. She was a great example of the caliber of people who have worked so hard to make the hospital what it is today.

Perspective...

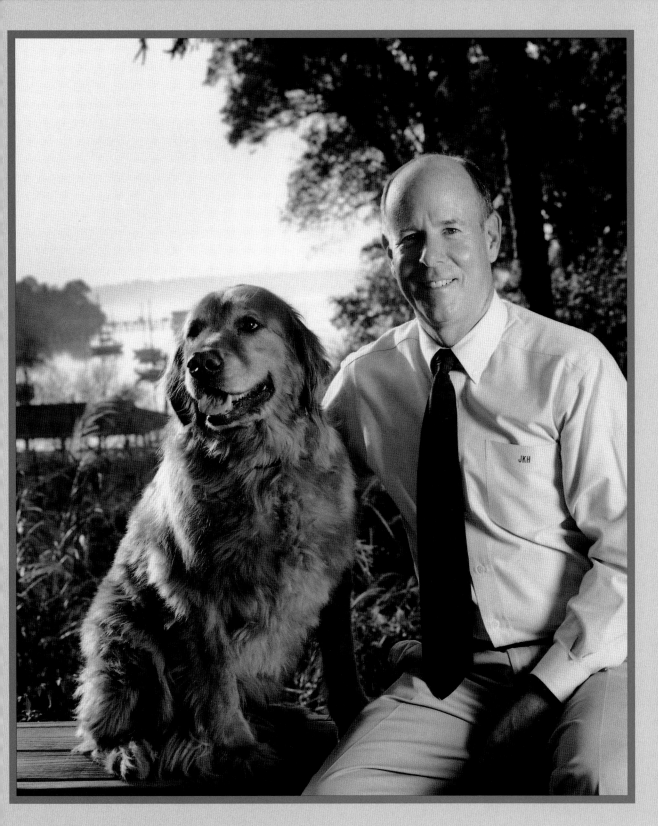

John "Jock" Hopkins

Lifelong Annapolitan

Board of Managers and Board of Trustees member, 1985-present

AAGHCS Board of Trustees president, 1991-1994

A s Anne Arundel Medical Center commemorated its 90th birthday in July 1992, there was ample cause for celebration. The downtown hospital continued to thrive, keeping pace with its Baltimore and Washington neighbors by offering ever more sophisticated diagnostic and treatment options. Medical Park was a success, too. The Outpatient Surgery Center and the Oncology Center which opened in 1989, were heavily utilized, with 3,713 outpatient surgeries and nearly 50 different community health programs in 1992. Plans were in place for a Women's Pavilion and a Medical Office Pavilion. Meanwhile, renovations to the aging downtown hospital were on the drawing board. The health system included an expanding network of outpatient facilities in areas that corresponded to local population growth, including three Anne Arundel Diagnostics centers and the Pathways substance abuse treatment facility, which opened in October 1992.

"We've been able to prosper partly because of where we're located—we're here by ourselves, in an affluent area. Plus, we've attracted a superior medical staff and extensive community support. We've been lucky, but we've also made our own luck."

John K. "Jock" Hopkins
AAGHCS/AAMC Board of Trustees Chair, 1991-1994

The county population was close to 450,000 and growing daily. Despite the incursion of managed care, the total number of hospital patients was on the rise, due to population growth and the increasing number of patients who traveled to the medical center from outlying areas. Still, with reduced occupancy, insurance company denials and payment delays, strict financial control of the $93 million operating budget became more important than ever.

Even with mounting marketplace pressures, in 1992 Anne Arundel Medical Center ranked among the 10 most efficient hospitals in Maryland, charging an average of 5.6 percent less per patient stay than other hospitals. In July 1992, the hospital reported $5,648,000 excess revenue over expenses, well above the meager margins of the 1980s. Clearly, hospital leaders were in firm control of finances.

At the helm was a talented team of professionally trained administrators—Carl A. "Chuck" Brunetto and Martin L. "Chip" Doordan. Together they demonstrated impressive staying power in an industry in which the average tenure of a hospital CEO was less than five years. And together they had the experience and community support to help them stay the course and chart the future, backed by boards that shared their commitment and vision. As important, they had the support of a 300-member medical staff and the backing of some 1,800 dedicated employees, many of whom had served the hospital for decades, and an 800-member Auxiliary.

"We've worked together so long that we know what each other is thinking."

Carl A. "Chuck" Brunetto
AAGHCS President, 1988-1994

"We always agree about the future direction for this health system."

Martin L. "Chip" Doordan
AAHS President, 1994-present

Rebecca Clatanoff accepts a plaque from John "Jock" Hopkins, chairman of the AAGHCS board (left), and Carl "Chuck" Brunetto, AAGHCS president, on Founder's Day, 1992. At this event, Mrs. Clatanoff learned that the new women's hospital would be named in her honor.

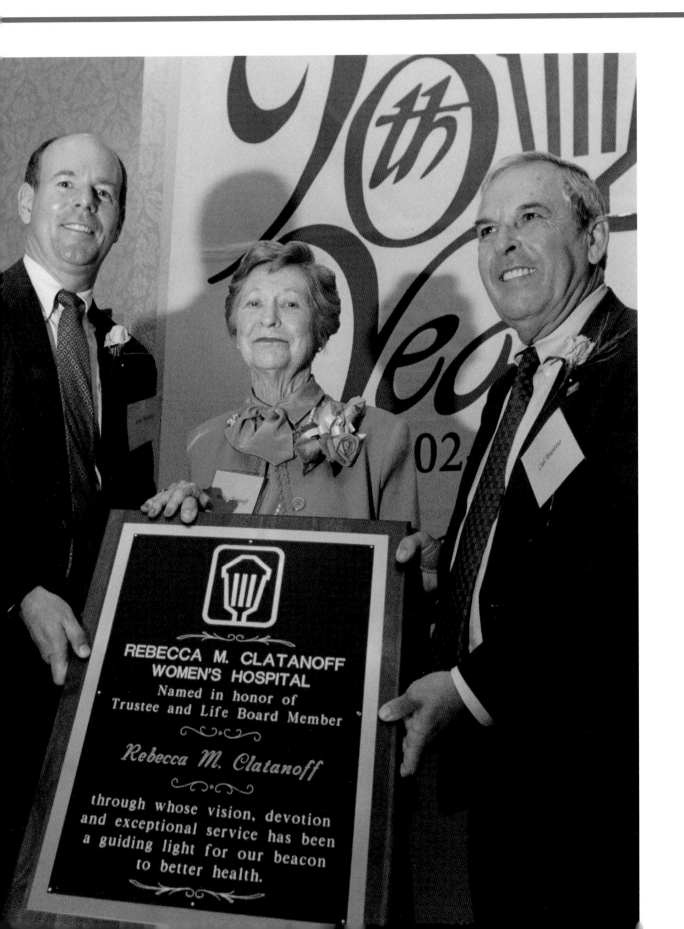

REBECCA M. CLATANOFF
WOMEN'S HOSPITAL
Named in honor of
Trustee and Life Board Member

Rebecca M. Clatanoff

through whose vision, devotion
and exceptional service has been
a guiding light for our beacon
to better health.

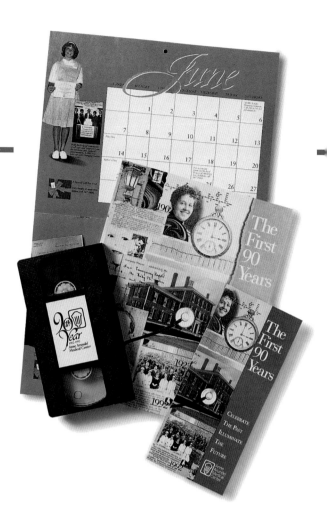

Undoubtedly, major change was on the horizon as the hospital approached its centennial. No more growth was possible at the 4.5-acre downtown site, plus renovation costs to the aging hospital were prohibitive. The site was limited by building and zoning restrictions and parking constraints. By contrast, the 60-acre Medical Park campus was more centrally located to future population centers, conveniently accessible to major roads and had ample room to grow. Hospital leaders projected that a new hospital would be necessary some 20 years hence.

"The acquisition of Medical Park was very fortunate. We were in the right place at the right time. It was meant to be this way."

Carl A. "Chuck" Brunetto
AAHS President, 1988-1994

In the interim, plans moved forward for the next phase of construction at Medical Park—the Women's Pavilion and the Medical Office Pavilion. The intent was to move high-volume, short-stay maternity services to Medical Park and provide space for physicians' offices. At the same time, the move provided space downtown to upgrade services.

The first step was to marshal the required financial resources. In March 1993, hospital leaders submitted a bond request for just over $73 million to cover costs of the new construction at Medical Park, the downtown hospital renovation and new capital equipment, and to pay off other debts.

Under the leadership of Lisa Hillman, executive director of the AAMC Foundation, the Foundation established the "Celebrate the Future" capital campaign. Chaired by local resident and business owner George Benson,

the Foundation set an initial goal of $6.6 million, later raising the goal to $8.6 million. The Auxiliary registered an early lead, pledging to raise $2 million by 1996. Anne Arundel County also participated, pledging $600,000. The medical staff raised $900,000 from among its ranks and employees contributed another $350,000.

"It was very gratifying to see the total commitment of the community, the Auxiliary, the hospital employees and the medical staff. It was wonderful to see what we all worked on finally come to fruition."

George Benson
"Celebrate the Future" Capital Campaign Chair

The money was to support both the old hospital and the new Women's Pavilion, to be called the Rebecca M. Clatanoff Pavilion in honor of the long-time volunteer, fundraiser, board member and hospital champion. Every member of the hospital family responded enthusiastically to the name choice, which honored a wonderful woman and fueled fundraising efforts.

Construction began in earnest in August 1993. Both pavilions were designed by Baltimore-based RTKL and built by J. Vinton Schafer & Sons of Baltimore, fitting into the existing landscape of pavilions. Project manager Carolyn Core, vice president of corporate services, and others traveled with key staff members to at least five different facilities, as far away as California, taking detailed notes and collecting ideas for the best possible obstetric facility. The aim was to provide the latest technology in a luxurious, patient-friendly, hotel-like setting.

The downtown hospital continued to add services, including a $3 million cardiac catheterization lab that opened in February 1993 and served as a valuable addition to the hospital's highly acclaimed coronary care unit and cardiac rehabilitation program. During the same time, maternity services were enhanced and the hospital's first critical care nursery opened. Oncology services also flourished, with new clinical pathways to improve care for patients with breast and prostate cancers and a long-range plan that focused on cancer prevention, early detection and comprehensive treatment. In a show of support, a group of area women established the "Stepping Out for Breast Cancer" program to raise funds for women with special needs.

The health system stayed true to its mission by continuing to reach out to the community. In 1994, the Outreach Clinic at the Lighthouse Shelter, staffed by volunteer physicians and nurses from the hospital, began to provide

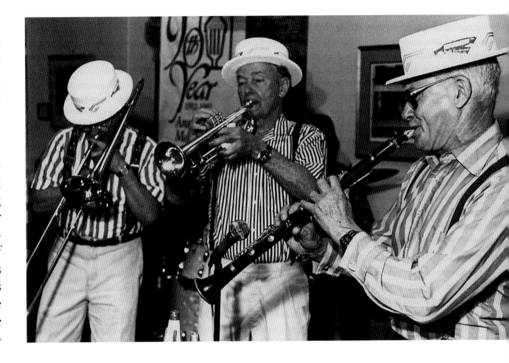

free medical services to uninsured residents. Soon after, the hospital received a $81,330 Domestic Violence grant from the state Department of Health and Mental Hygiene's Office of Health Promotion to establish a prototype to assist victims of domestic violence who came into the hospital's emergency department.

Effective management required leaders to allocate limited dollars carefully. Accordingly, the hospital closed its inpatient psychiatric unit in 1993 due to underutilization. Pathways faced dire financial straits, as insurers increasingly refused to cover costs for substance abuse programs. But Mr. Brunetto and Mr. Doordan, with support from the board, were committed to keeping Pathways open, noting that substance abuse was the number one problem in the county and it was the hospital's responsibility to meet the challenge.

And the band played on at AAMC's 90th birthday celebration in July 1992.

139

The AAMC Auxiliary celebrated its 50th year of service in 1994. Annual fundraisers included the Pink Lady Ball and many other activities.

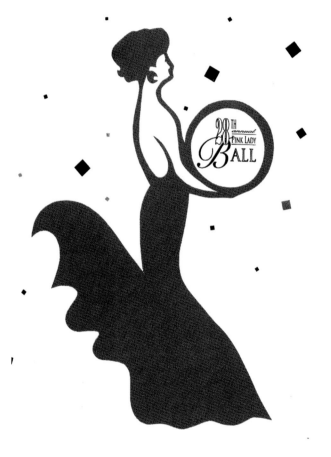

The health system continued to shore up its infrastructure outside the hospital walls, capitalizing on its positive cash flow. In 1994, a new Anne Arundel Diagnostics opened in Kent Island, extending the hospital's reach across the Chesapeake Bay Bridge to serve an ever-broadening geographic area.

As the health system expanded, it came time to simplify governance. In 1994, the Anne Arundel General Health Care Systems (AAGHCS) Board of Trustees and the Anne Arundel Medical Center Board of Directors merged to streamline operations, after just six years as separate entities. At the same time,

the health system's name was shortened to Anne Arundel Health System, Inc. (AAHS). These changes reflected the maturation of the health system.

The merged board also signaled a shift in the long-time management structure. Mr. Brunetto had suffered a heart attack in 1990, followed by surgery in 1991 and a lengthy recovery. Piece by piece, he turned over day-to-day operations to Mr. Doordan, his second in command, who became executive vice president of AAGHCS in 1993. Mr. Brunetto assumed the role of president emeritus and Mr. Doordan became president and chief executive officer of Anne Arundel Health System. A near-seamless "changing of the guard" had taken place.

Notably, the Auxiliary celebrated its 50th birthday in February 1994 and went on to sponsor the first Nordstrom Fashion Show and the 29th Pink Lady Ball that same year. The initial charter group had 20 members; by 1994, there were 909 members, 20 of them men. The Auxiliary had raised $6.5 million in 50 years. Members donated nearly 75,000 hours of service each year, serving in virtually every area of the hospital, managing the Clothes Box since 1952 and operating the Gift Shop and the Snack Bars, as well as hosting yearly book sales, jewelry sales and special events. In 1995, the Auxiliary opened its first "Lights on the Bay," an illuminated holiday display at Sandy Point State Park.

"Everyone is so pleased with Anne Arundel Medical Center and what it offers the community that it's natural that people gravitate toward joining the Auxiliary."

Barbara Ray
Auxiliary President, 1998-2000

The mid-1990s saw a lot of growth as hospital leaders pursued activity on multiple fronts. On January 31, 1995, a hospital pharmacist mistakenly filled syringes with morphine instead of heparin, which affected three infants in the new critical care nursery. It took several days to track down the source of the infants' distress. To compound matters, the hospital discovered that the pharmacist's license had expired. In its candor, the hospital shared this news with the public and made national headlines.

The hospital shut down the nursery temporarily, accepted the pharmacist's resignation and established new safety precautions. The Joint Commission for Accreditation of Healthcare Organizations (JCAHO) imposed "conditional" status in April, only to reinstate full accreditation in August.

> *"Anne Arundel Medical Center has always been known as an outstanding medical institution with a caring staff and a record of impeccable attention to detail. When its officials announced that the morphine found in three babies got there through carelessness, we're sure no one felt worse than the proud employees of AAMC, who strive for professional excellence."*
>
> *The Capital*
> February 19, 1995

Putting the pharmacy incident behind them, the hospital's management structure continued to evolve to better meet emerging needs. In October 1995, Carl Schindelar joined the team as chief operating officer. Dr. Jon Lowe left his position as medical director in 1995 to return to private practice and head the

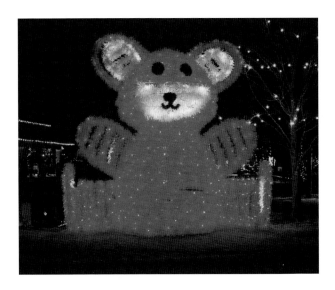

A giant teddy bear was a favorite at AAMC's illuminated holiday display, "Lights on the Bay," at Sandy Point State Park.

Community Wellness Initiative. He was replaced briefly by Dr. Jack Lord, who also had held the position in the early 1990s. Dr. Tony Greer took the helm in 1996, followed by Dr. Joseph Moser.

Modelcare 2000, a hospital initiative led by medical staff members and clinical administrators, established clinical initiatives in medicine, surgery, oncology, women's and children's services and wellness. Medical staff officers also began to receive compensation for their duties, as did physicians who served as medical directors of the hospital's clinical initiatives. Taken as a whole, these moves compensated doctors for the time they spent working on the hospital's behalf and served to continue to attract the highest caliber of physicians to these important positions.

Physicians definitely felt the managed-care pinch. In the mid-1990s, the board created a for-profit entity called Anne Arundel Health Care Enterprises to partner with physicians and stave off marketplace pressures. Attempts to form a Physician-Hospital Organization (PHO) were scrapped and a multi-specialty primary care group, called Health First, functioned for only a year. Similarly, physicians' efforts to work with national practice management companies failed and the hospital stepped in to ease pressure on some doctors so they were not forced to leave the area.

One plan to relieve pressure on physicians did work out well. In 1998, Anne Arundel Medical Center was one of the first hospitals in Maryland to bring in full-time pediatric hospitalists to help physicians under a contract with the University of Maryland Medical System. The program was a rousing success, and the medical center added hospitalists to oversee the care of adult patients that same year.

September 1995 was a hallmark month for the burgeoning medical center, marking the first time for inpatients at a second campus. The Rebecca M. Clatanoff Pavilion opened to great public fanfare, with nearly 6,000 people on hand to celebrate and tour the new facility.

The night before the facility opened, Lisa Hillman and Carolyn Core walked through the new facility to make sure everything was in place. Each had played a major role—Mrs. Hillman led the Foundation's successful drive; Mrs. Core oversaw each detail of construction. They walked through the eerily quiet pavilion, reflecting with pride on a job well done and thinking of the future generations of Annapolitans to be born in the new facility, beginning in just hours. These were the last moments of silence.

The Clatanoff Pavilion consolidated maternity, gynecology and women's diagnostics in a $28 million, three-story, 118,000-square-foot facility. The 22 labor/delivery/recovery/postpartum rooms filled up quickly with expec-

tant mothers anxious to experience the luxurious new facilities with state-of-the-art technology and a neonatal critical care unit. The pavilion also included the Breast Center, one of the region's first integrated breast care programs, and the Honor Roll of Women, a wall plaque that honored community women and raised money for women's health programs. Pediatric services moved to the pavilion in 1998.

"Our volume started to escalate right away and has increased 8-12 percent a year. Our goal has been to keep women and children in this community for their health care. Our challenge is to provide the best services we can."

Karen Peddicord, R.N., Ph.D.
AAMC Clinical Administrator
Women's and Children's Services

On September 14, the first baby born at the new facility was the son of John and Carol Frazer; Carol was an exercise physiologist at the hospital's cardiac rehabilitation service. The last baby at the downtown hospital was born to Tracy Watson and Lester Spicer that same day.

In 1995, the hospital anticipated 3,000 births, with expectations to grow to 4,000 by the year 2000. In fact, before the Clatanoff Pavilion even opened, a $3.5 million, 22,000-square-foot expansion plan already was underway to build out the third floor to accommodate 48-hour stays, recently mandated by the Maryland Legislature. In the interim, the hospital had to move gynecologic surgery patients back downtown to accommodate longer maternity stays at the new pavilion.

The Medical Office Pavilion also opened in

September 1995 and was a success from the outset. This project was a venture of Pavilion Park, Inc., a wholly-owned, for-profit subsidiary of Anne Arundel Real Estate Holding Company. The five-story, 75,000-square-foot facility opened with 100 percent of its offices under lease. As a busy medical office hub, it helped acquaint area residents with the new Medical Park site.

Continuing the tradition of naming new facilities for important members of the community, Medical Park was renamed the Carl A. Brunetto Medical Park in honor of the hospital's longtime administrator, who had retired in 1994 after 35 years with the health system.

The Outpatient Surgery Pavilion was formally renamed the Richard I. Edwards Pavilion in honor of Mr. Edwards, a long-time county resident and business owner, for his generous $1 million lifetime gift to the hospital.

"It's a great honor to have my name on the Medical Park sign, but under my name there should be 100 other names—the doctors who participated, the administrative staff who put in so much hard work, the community who raised the money to make it possible."

Carl A. "Chuck" Brunetto
AAHS President, 1988-1994

The Clatanoff Pavilion opened with much fanfare in September 1995, and quickly got down to the business of welcoming the next generation of Annapolitans.

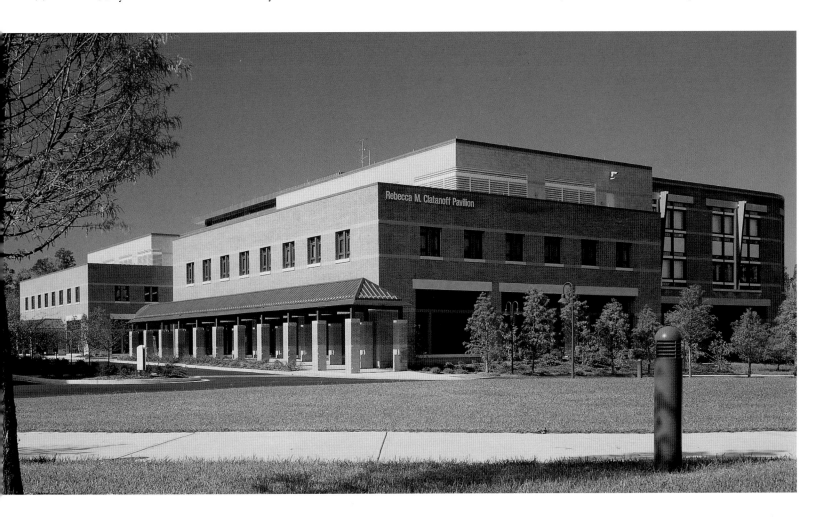

As they contemplated the future, hospital leaders considered strategies to best position the hospital to achieve its goals. Throughout the nation, hospitals banded together to respond to financial pressures. Although the medical center remained profitable, administrators had to contend with the realities of an aging hospital and a growing community. A partnership could offer the opportunity to increase services and reduce operating costs. On the other hand, it could lead to decreased autonomy. Hospital leaders decided to remain open to the idea, but proceed cautiously.

In September 1995, the same month that saw the opening of the Clatanoff and Medical Office Pavilions, the board approved a study to consider an affiliation with its Glen Burnie neighbor, North Arundel Hospital. After a series of talks and careful consideration over 10 months, both parties agreed to terminate affiliation discussions in July 1996. The board minutes noted that "remaining separate orga-nizations will best serve the greater Anne Arundel County area." In the final analysis, Anne Arundel Health System chose to remain independent.

In February 1997, the board formed a Networking Steering Committee to explore other potential affiliations. Through the rest of the year and into 1998, the board invited Helix Health/Medlantic Healthcare Group (later to become MedStar Health), the University of Maryland Medical System, Johns Hopkins Health System and Dimensions Health System to make presentations. All expressed great interest in collaborating with Anne Arundel Health System. Once again, the board decided to stay independent and make its own destiny.

The management team also remained open to limited affiliations with nearby health providers that could best respond to the community's needs. In fall 1997, the hospital entered into an agreement with the University

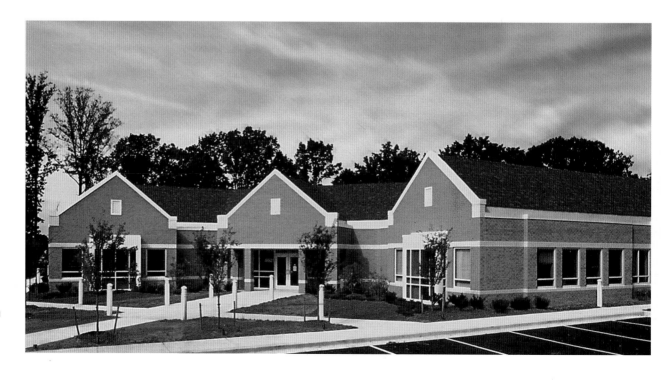

AAMC physicians worked alongside University of Maryland Medical Center specialists at Shipley's Choice Medical Park in Millersville, which opened in 1997. This extended AAMC's reach outside of Annapolis.

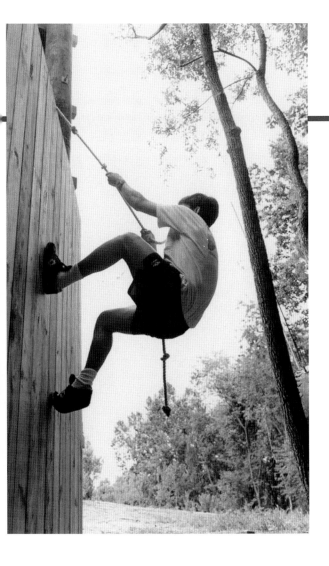

of Maryland Medical System in which local health care providers worked alongside UMMS specialists at Shipley's Choice Medical Park in Millersville.

"We felt it was important to explore alternatives, build relationships and remain flexible. In the end, we decided to pursue affiliations on a case-by-case basis where it made the most sense to partner."

Martin L. "Chip" Doordan
AAHS President

Even while neighboring health systems came courting, hospital leaders made plans for the future. Increasingly, the health system operated at two sites, duplicat-

ing security, food service, radiology and labwork downtown and at Medical Park. The two sites were a scant 2.8 miles apart, but they might as well have been in separate universes.

Immediately after the Clatanoff Pavilion opened in 1995, an extensive renovation to completely revamp the fourth floor of the downtown hospital was scheduled to begin. The mechanical and electrical infrastructure needed updating and patient care units also needed attention. But three days before construction was slated to start, hospital leaders called a halt to the project because the renovation did not improve patient care or facilitate the addition of more services. Instead, they reasoned, the money might be better spent on a new hospital.

It came down to a simple financial equation. It was expensive to duplicate services at two sites and if a consolidation netted $4 million in annual savings, that money could be used to service the debt for the new hospital. Planners determined that the numbers supported the decision to build a replacement hospital.

With the board, the administration and the medical staff firmly aligned, talk turned to plans for a new Acute Care Pavilion at Medical Park, a move that had loomed for years. The pieces fell into place quickly, although nearly 10 years ahead of schedule. The downtown facility was overtaxed and medicine continued to change rapidly, requiring updated facilities and new technologies.

"It was actually a fairly quick discussion, but it had taken years to get to that point. There were a series of decisions—Can we afford it?

Up to the challenge, a young wall climber tests his abilities at Pathways, a nonprofit substance abuse treatment program for adolescents and young adults. The 40-bed facility opened in 1992 as a cooperative venture of AAMC, the county and state.

Enthusiastic AAMC employees cheer as they celebrate their contribution to the "A New Century of Caring" capital campaign.

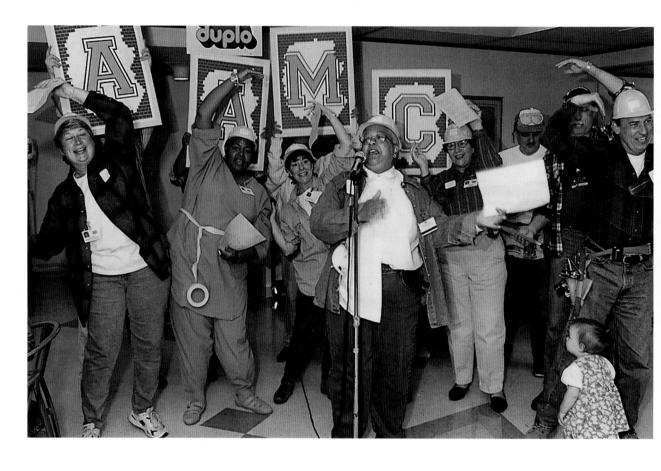

Can we raise the money? What should we do about the downtown facility? So many other decisions had to be made along the way, that it was almost anticlimactic. There was just a sense of relief."

John K. "Jock" Hopkins
AAHS Board of Trustees member, 1985-present

On October 31, 1996, the board voted to endorse the concept of consolidating inpatient facilities at Medical Park to improve patient care, access and cost. The carefully crafted motion had three parts—begin preliminary planning and design of a new facility, including financial feasibility and coordination with regulatory agencies; focus on city

concerns about the use of the downtown site and provision of future health services for residents, businesses and visitors; and communicate with all affected groups, providing opportunities for community input.

"It's now official: AAMC leaving city."

Headline in *The Capital*, November 5, 1996

Hospital officials talked to city and county officials the week before the board's vote. Anne Arundel Medical Center received state approval of an exemption from a Certificate of Need review because the new facility was a replacement hospital. A Consolidation Task Force oversaw the process, involving trustees, medical staff leaders and senior management.

THERE IS AN INCLUSIVE CULTURE HERE. WE WANTED EVERYONE TO FEEL
A SENSE OF OWNERSHIP IN THE NEW HOSPITAL. HUNDREDS OF PEOPLE
WERE INVOLVED IN DEVELOPING THE CONCEPT.

CAROLYN CORE, AAHS VICE PRESIDENT OF CORPORATE SERVICES

That same month, the administrative offices moved to Medical Park, a sign of things to come.

The medical staff was more than enthusiastic. They recognized the limitations of renovation and were excited about the possibilities for a brand new facility with the latest medical and information technology. When Mr. Doordan announced the pending move at a medical staff meeting, he was rewarded with a standing ovation.

"What we have is an opportunity to conceptualize and plan for health care into the next century, potentially to design a model health care facility that serves real needs, that builds community pride and that will stand for future generations."

Martin L. "Chip" Doordan
AAHS President
Letter to medical staff and employees
November 1, 1996

Building on her success with the recent construction at Medical Park, Carolyn Core was again named project manager. Dennis Curl, vice president of property development, also played a key role. Charles "Charlie" Steele functioned as "clerk of the works", overseeing the day-to-day details of the construction process. Wheeler, Goodman & Masek of Annapolis was named architect and J. Vinton Schafer & Sons of Baltimore was selected as construction manager. Hamilton KSA coordinated space planning. Over the life of the project, scores of consultants participated in different aspects of the development.

Chief architect Chuck Goodman listened to all the input about the shape the new hospital

should take, and added a good measure of his own ideas. In particular, he envisioned a hospital that would meet the emotional and spiritual needs of patients and families, while still providing top-notch medical care.

Plans for the new Acute Care Pavilion were time-consuming and enlightening. Once again, hospital leaders visited hospitals around the nation to find the best ideas and avoid the pitfalls. Of particular interest was a new hospital in Celebration, Florida that emphasized customer service. And, once again, Lisa Hillman and the Foundation made plans for a capital campaign to raise money to build the new hospital, which planners budgeted at $65-70 million.

The Consolidation Task Force held more than 100 meetings involving physicians, employees and community members to elicit ideas. The result was "Hopes, Dreams & Aspirations for the New Hospital," a simple one-page document that set overall direction, calling for a hospital that was patient-sensitive, cost-efficient, user-friendly, community health-focused, outpatient-oriented, high-tech with high-touch, and home for clinical centers of excellence.

The hospital also conducted a community survey to determine which factors were most important to area residents. A convenient, central location topped the list, followed, not surprisingly, by plentiful parking. Other factors important to the public were private rooms, family spaces and a larger, more efficient emergency department.

To provide an ongoing source of revenue, Anne Arundel Health System entered into an agreement with Constellation Real Estate Group, Inc. in 1996 to develop a 28-acre site across the street from Medical Park. This site was part of the health system's original purchase in 1984. The health system retained ownership of the land and Constellation assumed responsibility for developing the property, called Annapolis Exchange. Profits from the development would be shared between Anne Arundel Health System and Constellation, generating a future income to the health system. Constellation opened a 120,000-square-foot general office building in 2001.

"The hospital's expansion fits the needs of the community. It's a reflection of the increasing size and sophistication of the Annapolis area."

Philip Merrill
Chairman and Publisher, *The Capital*

As plans for the new Acute Care Pavilion took shape, talk turned to what to do with the old hospital, which was a beloved mainstay of downtown Annapolis. In spring 1997, the hospital formed a 15-member Site Re-use Advisory Committee, chaired by board members Becki Kurdle and April Moses and made up of representatives of the county, city, state, health system and neighborhood constituencies. The committee met for two years to develop criteria to guide the board in the sale of the property. The criteria for potential buyer/developers were compatibility with the neighborhood, economic impact, parking/traffic impact, design, community acceptance, value to the hospital, public amenity, tax benefit to the city and preservation of historic buildings.

"The process was inclusive of the people who would be affected by the hospital's move. We had no preconceived notions going in. The final decisions we made were reflective of the community as a whole."

Florence "Becki" Kurdle
Site Re-use Advisory Committee Co-chair
AAHS Board of Trustees Chair, 1997-99

Several factors helped ease residents' concerns about the transition ahead. The move to Medical Park had been gradual, which helped residents get used to the idea of a new health care hub. Also, hospital leaders kept their pledge to involve the community in determining the future use of the downtown hospital campus with a series of community meetings, and looked into ways to provide health care services downtown. Finally, it was difficult to contain the natural enthusiasm engendered by the possibilities of an all-new hospital.

In fall 1997, hospital leaders unveiled plans for the new Acute Care Pavilion at the annual association meeting. The emphasis was on patient-oriented, family-centered care, bringing technology to patients' bedsides in a hotel-like setting.

The site plan showed a six-story, 250,000-square-foot structure situated at the east end of the Medical Park complex. The number of beds in the new hospital was based on 12 months of average daily occupancy data, changing slightly over the life of the project. At the start, plans called for 147 private patient rooms, including an 18-bed critical care unit. The Clatanoff Pavilion housed 64 more rooms for obstetric, gynecologic and pediatric patients. The new hospital also included 10 surgical suites for inpatient and outpatient surgeries; adjacent procedure rooms for catheterization, endoscopy and interventional radiology; centralized diagnostics for easy access; a state-of-the-art emergency department with a helipad; and a 700-car adjacent garage for patient and visitors.

Throughout, there was a focus on efficiency, with the incorporation of the latest medical and information technology. As important, every effort was made to ensure that the facility was patient friendly, with private rooms, family areas, healing gardens and a nature theme.

"Our goal is to create a patient-sensitive, cost-efficient hospital with state-of-the-art technology. But what's behind the walls is just as important. We're adding the most up-to-date technology and infrastructure."

Dennis Curl
AAHS Vice President of
Property Development

Attention quickly turned to fundraising for the new hospital, starting in fall 1997. Building on the success of the Clatanoff Pavilion fundraising campaign, the board turned to the AAMC Foundation to spearhead the largest capital campaign in the area. Initial plans called for a community drive to raise $10 million; fundraisers dared to hope that the figure could go as high as $15 million. Hillard Donner, a long-time Annapolis resident, local business owner and chairman of the Foundation board, amazed fundraisers—and fellow Annapolitans—with a stunning $1 million pledge in October 1997. The "A New Century of Caring" capital campaign was off and running, with Mr. Donner as chairman. The Community Health Pavilion was renamed the Rose and Joseph Donner Pavilion for Mr. Donner's parents, in honor of his generosity.

The Auxiliary stepped up to the plate with a whopping $2.5 million commitment. Anne Arundel County made good on its promise to support the new hospital with a record-breaking $2 million commitment. At the outset, hospital employees pledged more than $800,000 and physicians raised more than $900,000. In July 1998, Anne Arundel Health System applied for a bond issue of nearly $70 million to build the new hospital.

"The hospital has been here for nearly 100 years and has been a mainstay of the community. They needed a catalyst from the county government to help them;

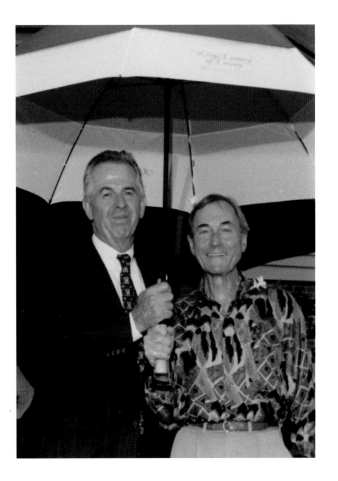

All smiles on a rainy day, AAMC President Martin "Chip" Doordan (left) and "A New Century of Caring" Capital Campaign Chair Hillard Donner provided inspirational leadership for the fundraising venture.

how could we not give them the financial help they needed? After all, the hospital has always displayed great generosity to the community. This is one of the better things I did during my time in office."

John Gary, Jr.
Anne Arundel County Executive, 1994-1998

The community helped out in ways large and small. A fourth grader, the daughter of a hospital employee, sent in $20 she earned through the sale of bookmarks. Local businesses threw their support behind the effort, too—banks made contributions, as did many area businesses. The Auxiliary published a cookbook, *A Feast of Memories*, in 1998 and donated the proceeds to a chapel fund for the new hospital, plus reinstituted the tradition of the annual Designer Show House. The Wayson family of south county, with roots in the community that go back 300 years,

pledged $1 million in February 1999, and the Medical Office Pavilion was renamed the Morgan B. and Martha O. Wayson Pavilion in honor of their grandparents. Based on its fundraising success, the AAMC Foundation also garnered a prestigious Kresge matching fund grant for $600,000, announced the day of groundbreaking ceremonies for the new hospital on December 16, 1998.

While hospital leaders made plans to build a new Acute Care Pavilion, they continued to add increasingly sophisticated services. Clinical planning was a two-way street, sometimes initiated by physicians and sometimes by administrators. The overriding plan was to consolidate programs and integrate services to deliver the best patient care, forming "centers of excellence." Whenever possible, leaders vowed to make use of local medical talent, recruiting specialists from elsewhere to bring new skills and fresh ideas when it made the most sense and

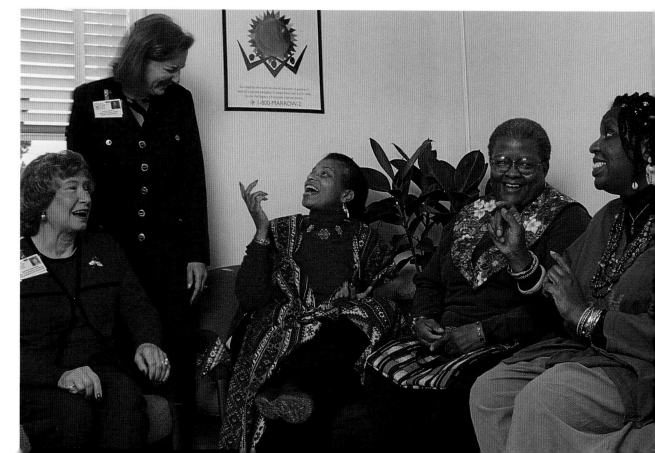

AAMC nutritionist Ann Caldwell, R.N. combines a nutrition class with an Annapolis Outreach Center holiday social. Enjoying the event are (left to right) Bea Carpenter, health screening technician; Caldwell; Faye Hunt-Anderson, R.N., outreach services coordinator; Carolyn White and Marilyn Jones-Thomas.

providing seed money for new practices when necessary.

"Becoming a regional medical center goes beyond expanding the system. It requires the ability to deliver specialty care close to home, so patients don't have to go to Baltimore or Washington. They can have confidence that we'll provide excellent care here."

Dr. Joseph D. Moser
AAHS Vice President of Medical Affairs

The Center for Joint Replacement was established in 1996, becoming the hospital's first true center of excellence, with a full line of services coordinated to improve results, reduce complications and speed recovery. The newly integrated approach to patient care netted impressive results. With the lowest charges in the region, demand increased 24 percent with 104 patients in the first four months of operation.

"I'm especially happy for the patients. It's been a good thing for them and it's revolutionized joint care in the United States. Our program is very well known nationally and internationally."

Dr. Marshall K. Steele III
Orthopedic surgeon
Medical Director, Surgical Services

To round out cardiac services, the hospital added electrophysiology and, later, ablation services to the cardiac catheterization lab. In 1998, the hospital expanded its critical care capability to meet the growing demand. The Spine Center opened, building on the same model of care that proved so successful for

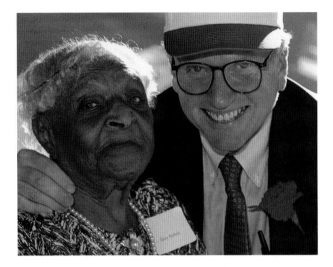

Daisy Nichols, 102, of Annapolis, poses with her surgeon, Dr. Marshall K. Steele III at the Joint Camp Reunion held for former joint replacement patients and their coaches in 1999. The Center for Joint Replacement won regional and national awards for excellence.

the Center for Joint Replacement. Other downtown additions included an outpatient pulmonary rehabilitation program, two new endoscopy suites and a Sleep Disorders Center.

Enhancements were underway at Medical Park, too. The Clatanoff Pavilion opened its third floor in May 1997 and gynecologic services moved to Medical Park for good. In November 1997, the state approved a Certificate of Need for a Level III+ neonatal intensive care unit with the technology and expertise to handle the most premature babies. Pediatrics moved to the second floor of the Clatanoff Pavilion in March 1998, occupying brand-new, child-friendly space.

Also at Medical Park, the outpatient surgery facility increased from four to six operating rooms to meet the explosive demand. The radiation oncology department added a state-of-the-art three-dimensional radiation treatment planning system in 1997 to improve cancer care. The hospital established a Diabetes Center, which was approved by the American Diabetes Association, to offer comprehensive diabetes education.

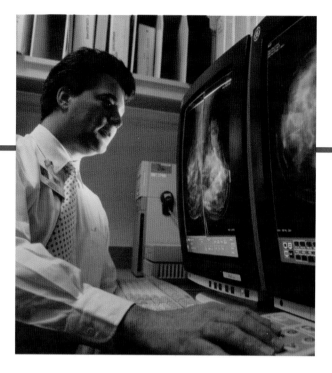

Dr. George W. Adams interprets a digital mammogram. AAHS offers comprehensive imaging services at Anne Arundel Diagnostics centers at eight locations around the region, linked by computers for efficiency.

At the same time, the health system continued its community outreach efforts. In 1996, the popular ASK-A-NURSE program was established, offering 24-hour interactive telephone service to community residents, with health information, physician referrals and community health program registration. In 1997, Anne Arundel Medical Center became one of the first hospitals in the state to establish its own web site, yet another way to reach out to residents. A new Wellness Van began traveling to health fairs and community events in 1998 to educate county residents about health issues and provide screenings.

Hospital leaders made good on their promise to maintain a health care presence in downtown Annapolis. The Annapolis Outreach Center, staffed by hospital volunteers, opened in 1998 to serve the health care needs of downtown residents. The new center was an outgrowth of the Lighthouse Shelter.

The health system continued to expand in every direction. In 1998, Anne Arundel Health System entered into a venture with Nighttime Pediatrics, a privately owned after-hours facility in Parole, providing services that allowed expansion to "Adult Care, Too!"

In October 1998, Anne Arundel Medical Center was thrilled to earn the Mercury Award

from America's Health Network and HCIA as the top hospital overall in the Baltimore region. Out of 23 hospitals, Anne Arundel Medical Center earned the coveted #1 position overall, achieving a score of 100 percent. Anne Arundel Medical Center also was #1 in cardiology, #2 in oncology and #4 in orthopedics, based on statistical measures of patient survival rates, complication rates and staffing ratio—in short, the measures that matter most to patients when they are selecting a hospital. The award proved that the hospital recognized the needs of the community and took steps to meet those needs.

The year ended on another high note, with the December 16, 1998, groundbreaking for the new Acute Care Pavilion. Some 600 officials were in attendance. Nearly 50 school-children, all wearing hardhats, gathered on the cold winter morning and formed a ring around the freshly dug hole to sing a song about the future. This simple gesture reminded attendees of the purpose—and the promise—behind the project that was about to begin in earnest. Within days, bulldozers quickly gathered and construction workers began site preparation work.

"This is the moment to expand our vision, to realize new possibilities and to go beyond what we can only imagine today."

Martin L. "Chip" Doordan
AAHS President
December 16, 1998

The next year started with a double financial hit. Maryland's Health Services Cost Review Commission (HSCRC) issued a 1 percent rate reduction per case, which further constrained the hospital operating budget and required strict financial oversight. And then the medical center agreed to pay Medicare $2.1 million to settle a home infusion payment issue; the amount was far more than what was mistakenly collected. Still, 1999 turned out to be one of the hospital's most successful years ever, with excess revenue of $16.2 million over expenses.

"We have a productivity system in place and we've managed our costs efficiently. Our financial health is directly tied to increasing patient admissions. And that is testimony to the confidence that our community has in this hospital."

George Blair
AAHS Vice President of Finance

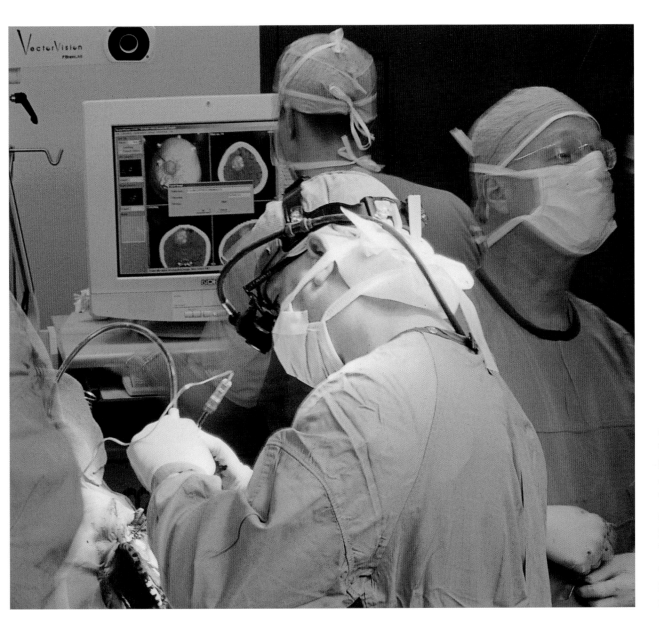

During a craniotomy, AAMC neurosurgeons work together. Dr. Clifford T. Solomon (center) uses Vector Vision-guided instruments to locate the tumor, while Dr. Thomas B. Ducker (right) accesses information on another monitor.

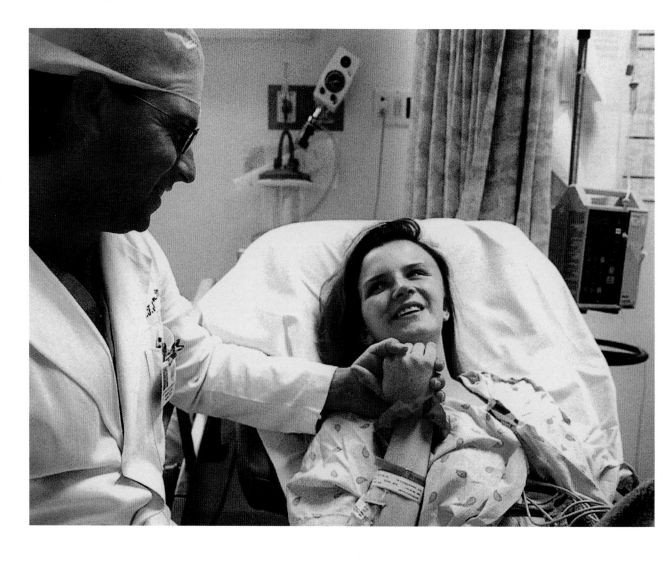

Neurosurgeon Dr. Clifford Solomon talks with Kelli Rigsbee after emergency surgery to stop bleeding in her brain. Both the patient and her unborn baby survived, beating the odds.

In January 1999, the hospital sent out 200 letters to potential buyers of the downtown site, followed by Requests for Proposals to 63 interested parties. Submitted proposals included projects for housing, assisted living, hotel, mixed use and office developments. Most were from Maryland and Virginia, but responses came from as far away as Illinois and Connecticut.

After reviewing 12 proposals and hearing presentations by four finalists, the board selected Virginia-based Madison Homes in September 1999 as the future owner/developer of the downtown site. Plans called for the new site to include a mixture of condominiums, townhomes, village homes and single-family homes, plus age-restricted (55+) condominiums to be constructed on Franklin, Shaw and Cathedral Streets. The new development was named Acton's Landing—a tribute to Richard Acton, an original Annapolis landowner—and included a waterfront park. The developers also offered to preserve the historic brick building on the corner of Franklin and Cathedral streets, with a potential for community use. The hospital decided to retain ownership of 51 Franklin Street and continue to house its financial operations department there. The final purchase price depended on the city's ultimate approval of the project.

"Overall, we felt it just fit. We looked at all the criteria from different aspects and when we added it all up, Madison Homes was the winner."

Martin L. "Chip" Doordan
AAHS President
The Capital, September 24, 1999

To house new ambulatory services and accommodate more physicians' offices, Pavilion Park made plans to build a six-story, 150,000-square-foot Ambulatory Health Pavilion—later named the Lesly and Pat Sajak Pavilion—with outpatient clinical services and physicians' offices. In June 1999, ground was broken for this new facility.

Work also began on an oncology business plan to create a cancer center to increase services for the area's cancer patients. The hospital continued to expand its cancer programs. In 1999, Anne Arundel Medical Center expanded its Breast Center, bringing together a team of excellent surgeons and oncologists and a director, Dr. Lorraine Tafra, to offer such innovations as sentinel node biopsy to determine the spread of cancer, plus all the most advanced radiation therapy and chemotherapy options. The Breast Center had been established in 1995, offering innovative surgery approaches by Dr. George E. Linhardt, Jr. and his associates, and one of the region's first Lymphedema Centers. Other new cancer treatment options included prostate seed implantation (also called brachytherapy), which used radioactive seeds to treat prostate tumors directly, and minimal-

ly invasive approaches to surgery whenever possible. That year, 971 new cancer patients were seen with a wide range of diagnoses.

"AAMC's Oncology Initiative continues to make significant strides in dealing with the needs of patients in our community who develop cancer, launching prevention programs and educating our community about this disease. These efforts will have a significant effect on the quality of life of residents of our community."

Dr. Stanley P. Watkins, Jr.
Medical Director of the Oncology Center
2000 Annual Report

In 1999, there was an explosion of new clinical services. A neurosurgery program was established and Vector Vision technology was added, consisting of a computerized navigational device that aids in delicate brain surgery. The hospital also was among the first in the area to offer laparoscopic spinal surgery, a less invasive approach to back surgery, and sophisticated retinal surgery to correct vision disorders. A Maternal-Fetal Medicine Program was added to tend to high-risk pregnancies. Vascular surgery services took off, with new surgeons and new techniques, supported by a vascular ultrasound lab. To improve patient care in every service, innovative pain management techniques were implemented.

"We've made an effort to keep up with emerging technologies so we can continually improve patient care."

Dr. Vernon R. Croft
Radiologist
AAMC Chairman of Medicine

Anne Arundel Medical Center had much to offer new physicians—a rapidly growing health system, a new hospital and easy access to academic centers in Baltimore and Washington, topped off by a great quality of life in Annapolis. It also had much to offer patients—excellent care, close to home. In 1999, the public relations department, under the direction of Martha Harlan, R.N., instituted an award-winning advertising campaign— Superior Care. Right Here. Right Now.— which integrated marketing and communications and highlighted its breast cancer, vascular and prostate services.

Construction continued apace at Medical Park, which celebrated its 10th anniversary in August 1999. The foundation for the new Acute Care Pavilion was in place and the building rapidly took shape. With the Lions Club support, the new helipad opened in October, and construction of the Ambulatory Health Pavilion proceeded on schedule.

For the time being, the downtown hospital still served as the center of the health system's acute care universe. The emergency department underwent much-needed renovation in 1999 and added a Fast Track to treat minor illnesses and injuries. The effort paid off and patient satisfaction increased dramatically. Similarly, many other areas of the hospital scored high in patient satisfaction.

Community health partnerships capitalized on the resources of local agencies to bring residents the programs they most wanted. In March 1999, Anne Arundel Medical Center and the Anne Arundel County Department of Health collaborated to reach out to children up to age 19 and pregnant mothers who are eligible for insurance covered under the Maryland Children's Health Insurance Program, passed by the Maryland Legislature in 1998.

In 1999, with so many irons in the fire, the health system decided to transfer its home health and hospice services to MedStar Health, to be operated by the Visiting Nurses Association of Washington, D.C. The service was too small to run efficiently, so administrators elected to focus on acute care, while making sure that county residents had access to home health care. The new service was called Anne Arundel Home Health and Hospice. In September 2001, hospice services were transferred to Hospice of the Chesapeake, in agreement with the medical center.

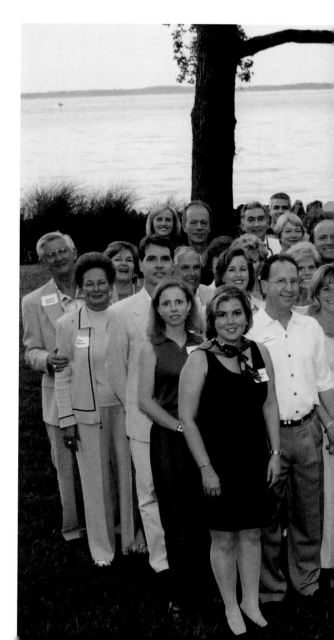

Guests Lesly and Pat Sajak (center) join campaign volunteers and AAMC staff at the home of Dr. Lou and Laurie Berman in the summer of 2000 to celebrate their fundraising success. The "A New Century of Caring" campaign went on to raise a record-breaking amount—nearly $22 million.

156

The year closed with another prestigious award. Anne Arundel Medical Center was named a Top 100 hospital in the nation for orthopedics by HCIA, a particular honor for its three-year-old Center for Joint Replacement. Patients also recognized the program's strength. Each year, a "Joint Camp" reunion was held for former patients, attracting as many as 700 celebrants.

As the 20th century drew to a close, the medical center was on the national map. It was firmly established as a regional medical center, drawing a large number of its patients from outside a 10-mile radius and offering increasingly sophisticated services and integrated centers of excellence.

The millennium dawned with nary a disruption. Around the world, people watched anxiously as computers switched from 1999 to 2000. When the original computer programs were written in the 1960s, computers were programmed to recognize just the last two digits of the year, so massive fixes were necessary to avert the dis-

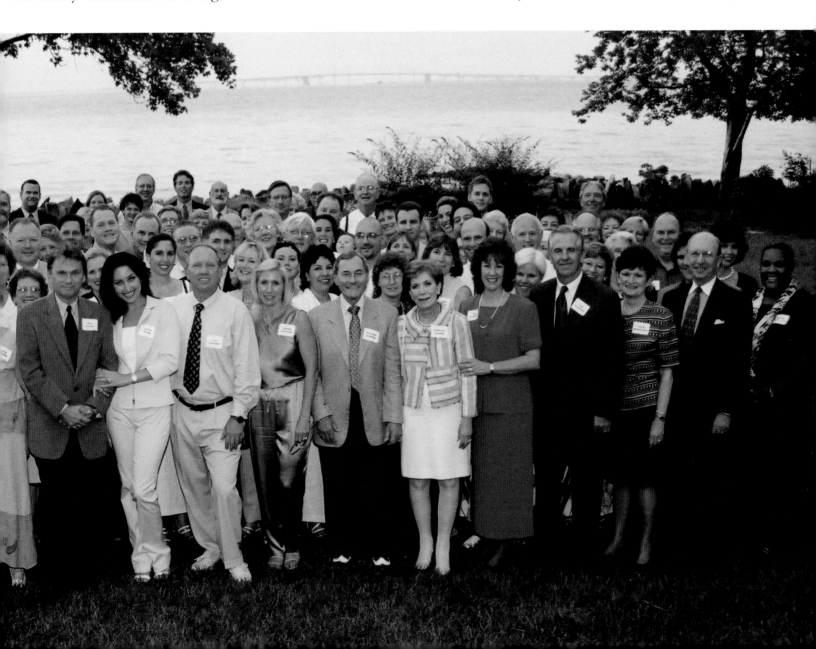

In 1997, AAMC was one of the first hospitals in the state to establish a web site.

To get the word out, AAMC produced integrated campaigns that informed the community about its sophisticated services and distributed *Vital Signs* to the community.

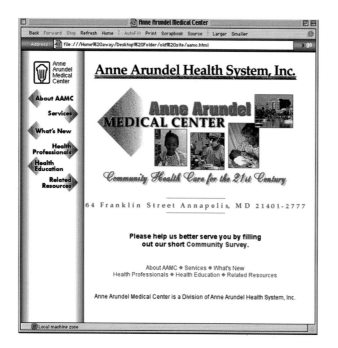

aster that could occur if computers misconstrued the new date to be 1900, rather than 2000.

After months of preparation that cost an estimated $1-2 million, the hospital's computers reset from 1999 to 2000 with no glitches. Senior staff members attended a pre-midnight gathering in the cafeteria. As the clock moved toward midnight, everyone assumed their posts to make sure the hospital continued to function normally. That day, eight babies were born, 143 patients visited the emergency department and 32 new patients were admitted to the hospital.

"As the New Year dawned, I climbed to the hospital garage roof to watch the fireworks over City Dock. I realized that the hospital we had known for nearly a century soon would be demolished. But I was excited about the new hospital and so proud of this community for making it happen."

Lisa Hillman
AAHS Vice President of Development
and Community Affairs

To celebrate the New Year and commemorate the changes underway, a new hospital logo was unveiled. It featured an updated beacon symbol, showing that the lamp had broken out of its box. The new form suggested the growth of the system and continued outreach to the community.

Business continued to boom—Anne Arundel Medical Center was the fastest growing hospital in the state. Inpatient admissions jumped 26.9 percent between 1995 and 2000. By 2000, inpatient admissions climbed to 18,648, with 50,929 emergency department visits. The hospital was the fourth busiest birthing facili-

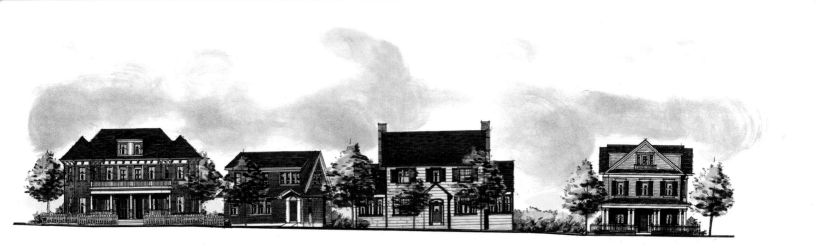

ty in the state, with 4,029 births. Surgery was up 12 percent, with 4,733 inpatient surgeries and 10,548 outpatient surgeries. The number and breadth of community health programs continued to grow tremendously through the years, and included screening services, integrative health programs and a popular "Health for the Whole Woman" series of lectures, for a total of 475 health care programs in fiscal year 2000 that drew 4,775 participants.

With heavy demand on its services, the hospital sought ways to cope with another national health care issue—the shortage of nurses and other health care providers. In February 2000, the hospital instituted a pay raise for all nurses involved in direct patient care—some 600 full- and part-time nurses. Human resources staff sought other ways to add manpower, including the use of agency help, creative recruiting measures, mentorship programs and cooperative arrangements with Anne Arundel Community College and Bowie State University, among others. The intent was to retain existing employees and attract some 60-80 additional nurses for the new hospital.

The new hospital took shape rapidly. On April 20, 2000 there was a topping-off party; the last beam was set to swing into place! Nearly 1,000 residents signed or placed a message on the metal girder, showing the depth of community support behind the hospital. Construction workers hoisted the beam as attendees cheered in appreciation. Over the life of the project, dozens of contracting companies were involved. Each day, about 300 workers were on site, representing many different specialties.

"Considering this is a design/build project, things have gone very smoothly. Because we're adapting as we go along, it requires active management and participation. A project like this has to be a team effort."

Charles "Charlie" Steele
Clerk of the Works

Heavy demand on the surgical facilities necessitated the addition of two operating rooms to the downtown hospital in 2000, converted from existing endoscopy suites. Correspondingly, the decision was made to add 27,000 square feet of space to the new hospital for additional operating and

Madison Homes was selected as the developer for the downtown site in 1999. Community members were actively involved in establishing criteria for the project.

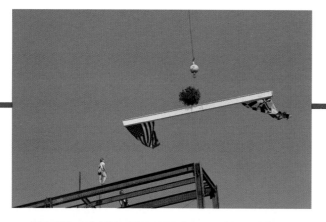

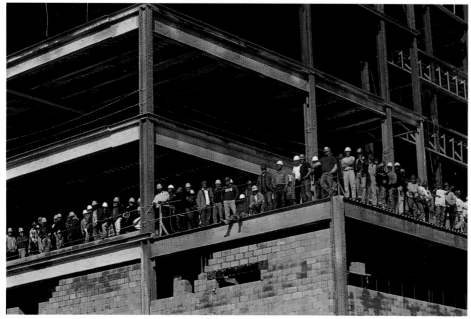

The last beam for the new hospital swung into place on April 20, 2000. Nearly 1,000 people signed the metal girder.

with outstanding results and lengths of stay just half that of other Maryland hospitals.

"Our neuroscience services bring together a team of specialists to offer patients all the most sophisticated services, close to home. Everything's right here and we're among the first in the region for many of the most innovative approaches."

Dr. Clifford T. Solomon
AAMC neurosurgeon

In recognition of the growing number of patients in Anne Arundel County and the excellence of care provided by the hospital, Kaiser Permanente signed a landmark agreement with Anne Arundel Health System in 2000 as a regional referral center for Kaiser members in the county. The medical center also was selected by the American Hospital Association to participate in a series of health fairs on Capitol Hill. It was one of only eight hospitals and one of three from Maryland.

Closer to its traditional base of operations, Anne Arundel Medical Center joined in a cooperative effort with the City of Annapolis and the Anne Arundel County Health Department to establish the Stanton Community Center, which opened in July in the old Stanton building that had served as a school for African-American children since 1900. The Annapolis Outreach Center moved its base of operations into the Stanton Community Center, offering residents access to specialists in dermatology, diabetes, gynecology and ophthalmology.

The hospital also continued to receive accolades for excellence. In July 2000, hospital staffers were delighted to find that Anne Arundel Medical Center was named to *U.S.*

procedure rooms. The 700-space parking garage opened in the spring, offering covered parking. At the same time, two new post-delivery rooms opened in the Clatanoff Pavilion, to handle the rapidly increasing number of births.

Hospital leaders continued to pursue efforts to offer the most advanced services to patients. A national center for minimally invasive abdominal aortic aneurysm surgery was established—with the expertise of vascular surgeons, interventional radiologists and cardiologists, and with Dr. John Martin as director—and served as a training site for other doctors. The hospital's team of neurosurgeons, led by Dr. Thomas Ducker, Dr. Clifford Solomon and Dr. Brian Sullivan, performed about 100 neurosurgery procedures in 2000,

News & World Report's "America's Best Hospitals" list in two categories—gynecology and respiratory diseases. It was one of just six hospitals in Maryland to make the list and one of very few community hospitals to earn a coveted slot on the top 50.

"What drew me to AAMC is the strategic vision this hospital has. I've been very impressed with the administration's relationship with the staff and the caliber of the medical staff. The level of community participation has really been outstanding. A hospital has to have all those factors in place to succeed."

Sharon Riley
AAHS Chief Operating Officer

Administrative changes were underway, too. Sharon Riley joined the system as chief operating officer in July 2000; Carl Schindelar left in August 1999 to head a Baltimore hospital. In September 2000, a longstanding provision in the bylaws that gave hospital association members voting rights to amend bylaws and elect board members was changed. In recent years, only a handful of community members attended the annual meeting in September, a dramatic reduction from the hundreds of attendees at contentious meetings during earlier decades. The rule was changed and the Board of Trustees gained the ability to change bylaws and elect new members who reflected the increasing diversity and specialization required to lead the health system into the next century.

The "A New Century of Caring" capital campaign met its updated goal of $20 million and went on to raise nearly $2 million more. This was more than twice the original goal and even the fundraising consultants were amazed. Later that year, the AAMC Foundation sponsored a much-deserved Thankathon, with phone calls to 700 donors thanking them for their support.

The Foundation next turned its attention to raising $2 million for the new Breast Center. The campaign got off to a rousing start in October with a $1 million donation from Lesly and Pat Sajak (the television personality who lives in Severna Park), followed by a generous gift from campaign chair Judy and Dr. Lamon Stewart. The Ambulatory Health Pavilion was named the Lesly and Pat Sajak Pavilion in honor of the Sajaks' $1 million contribution.

All phases of the construction of the Acute Care Pavilion were documented by regional media—from groundbreaking to a celebration of near completion by Martin "Chip" Doordan, AAHS president (left); Carolyn Core, vice president of corporate services; and Chuck Goodman, architect.

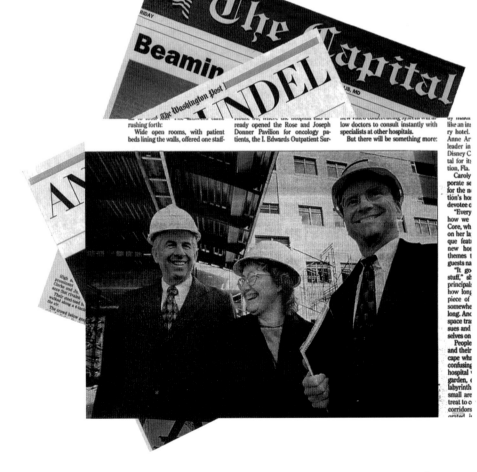

In 2000, the hospital's web site—www.aahs.org—was expanded to include on-line physician referral, health information and on-line giving capability. The Auxiliary implemented "The Baby Shop at AAMC," a web-based program that allows users to purchase flowers or gifts and the Auxiliary to raise money at the same time.

Clearly, Anne Arundel Health System was doing many things right. The medical center was one of only a handful of hospitals that remained independent after the turbulent 1990s. North Arundel Hospital was acquired by the University of Maryland Medical System in 2000. Johns Hopkins bought Howard County General Hospital in 1998. Helix Health and Medlantic Healthcare Group formally merged to create MedStar Health in 1999, with a total of seven hospitals in Baltimore and Washington by 2000.

By contrast, Anne Arundel Medical Center posted $13.4 million excess revenue over expenses in 2000, when 40 percent of hospitals in Maryland lost money. It expanded its regional service area to include some 600,000 residents. It was the county's fourth largest private employer with some 2,000 full- and part-time employees, supported by an active Auxiliary with more than 900 members who volunteered 82,000 hours a year. The medical staff increased 15 percent in the past year alone and numbered nearly 600 members.

As plans were made to move to the new Acute Care Pavilion in late 2001, a controversy erupted concerning Madison Homes, the developer selected to purchase and develop the site of the downtown hospital. One of its principal partners had been cited for questionable workmanship by tenants on several earlier projects and had

declared bankruptcy, newly incorporating the company under the name Madison Homes. Since that time, they had several successful projects, but local residents were concerned.

The hospital was caught unawares when the news broke late in 2000. The committee had conducted a background check of the current company and tenants of its projects, but had not uncovered the defunct business ventures. Hospital leaders quickly convened a community meeting to address concerns and reassure citizens. *The Capital* weighed in with an editorial, saying that it was the city's responsibility to ensure high-quality construction standards and the controversy subsided.

"We chose Madison Homes because they had the plan that best met the criteria established by our advisory group. They also demonstrated a sincere interest in working with the city to create a project to complement the neighborhood."

Florence "Becki" Kurdle
Site Re-use Advisory Committee Co-chair
AAHS Board of Trustees Member, 1991-2000

As people from further away began using Anne Arundel Medical Center, the health system continued to stretch its service area. It established a base of operations in Bowie, when AAMC Health Services-*Bowie* opened early in 2001, offering diagnostics and medical specialty services. The three-story 26,000-square-foot facility contained offices for some 80 physicians.

Other efforts were made to expand services. Plans were put into place to expand programs in gynecologic oncology, lung cancer and colorectal cancer. Further, the health system formed a partnership with Children's National

Medical Center in Washington, D.C. to provide round-the-clock pediatric hospitalists to staff the hospital's inpatient pediatric unit. The agreement left the door open for future sub-specialty services.

During the winter, hospital leaders testified before the Maryland Legislature in an attempt to change existing Certificate of Need statutes so the medical center could add open heart surgery to its growing list of services. They determined to continue this effort in future years.

In March 2001, the Sajak Pavilion officially opened. Some 1,200 guests attended the March 8 celebration in a large tent outside the new pavilion. The $25 million building contained a host of outpatient facilities, including the new Breast Center—with 7,000 square feet of space it was one of the largest such facilities in the nation, equipped with state-of-the-art, three-dimensional digital mammography technology. Also in the Sajak Pavilion were the Diabetes Center, the Vascular Institute, the Maryland Neurological Institute, AAMC Community Health and Wellness, Anne Arundel Diagnostics, the Clothes Box, administrative offices and doctors' offices. A four-level attached garage provided ample parking space as tenants moved in throughout 2001.

As the Acute Care Pavilion neared completion, planners were already hard at work on upcoming projects to further expand the health system. The health system's annual operating budget for 2002 was $220 million. The region continued to grow by leaps and bounds. Projections called for the hospital's service area to incorporate nearly 720,000 residents by 2004, including Anne Arundel County, parts of Prince George's County, and Queen Anne, Kent and Calvert counties. In fiscal year 2001, the hospital enjoyed a record

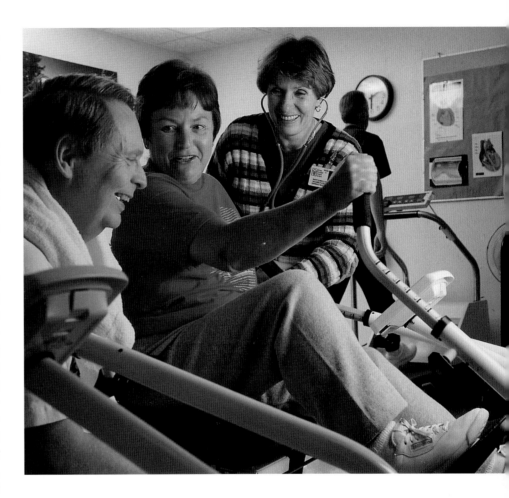

4,399 births and had the fourth highest annual volume in the state.

An outpatient cancer center was scheduled to begin construction in 2002 to handle the annual volume of some 11,000 cancer treatments. In June, the medical center received a $56,000 grant from the Susan G. Komen Foundation to establish a post-residency breast fellowship—one of a few hospitals in the nation to host such a program—which served as testimony to the excellence of care at the Breast Center.

The medical center leased space in a new medical office building under construction in

James Witt encourages patient Betty Malen (center) while Libby Vinson, R.N. takes Mrs. Malen's blood pressure. AAMC's cardiopulmonary rehab program uses education, exercise and support to help cardiac patients improve their cardiovascular function.

As AAMC approached its 100th birthday, the new Acute Care Pavilion neared completion. The hospital had emerged as a major regional medical center, earning national recognition for excellence.

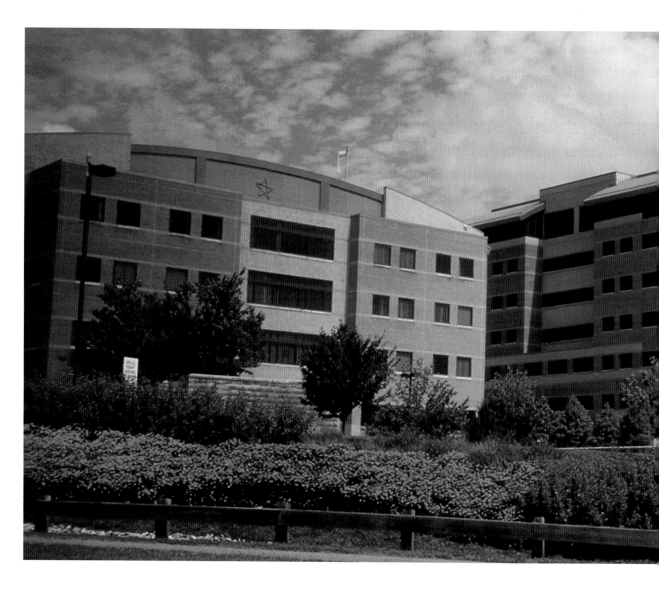

Gambrills—the Village at Waugh Chapel, slated to open in 2002—similar to the Bowie facility with physicians' offices, diagnostics and urgent care. That brought the number of Anne Arundel Diagnostics centers to eight; any resident of the region had no more than 5.5 miles to drive to get to the nearest facility.

Space was still available for future growth. There was discussion of perhaps a second acute care facility and garage adjacent to the new hospital. Similarly, space was still available for a second medical office and garage near the Sajak Pavilion.

Leaders already were planning for the next wave of programmatic and facilities growth to meet the needs of the expanding region. In December 2001, the board adopted Vision 2005, a strategic plan that addressed the growth of the health system after the medical center's move to Medical Park.

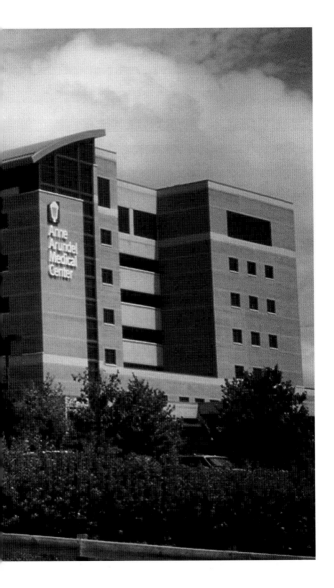

Wired Hospitals and Health Care Systems" in the nation, a tribute to its state-of-the-art information technology.

"We've set the stage for significant additional expansion. We've planted the seeds, expanded into new market areas, expanded our clinical capabilities and become a full-service regional medical center. I have a tremendous sense of pride in all the people here— the administration, the employees, the medical staff, the volunteers."

James F. McEneaney, Jr.
AAHS Board of Trustees Chair, 1999-present

In September, as the new hospital was nearing completion, disaster struck the United States. On the sunny Tuesday morning of September 11, the world stood still as terrorists attacked the World Trade Center and the Pentagon. Annapolitans quickly rose to the occasion. Several hundred residents showed up at the hospital that day, waiting in line for a chance to donate blood to help the victims. Many returned the next day, while others called for appointments in the weeks ahead. Meanwhile, hospital leaders joined county and state agencies in preparing a disaster plan for a new world order.

Throughout the year, local officials, community leaders, physicians, hospital employees, media members—anyone with an interest—took "hard hat tours" of the new Acute Care Pavilion. Every week, there was a new bit of progress and excitement continued to build. The hospital held its 99th birthday party on July 18, its last formal event at the downtown site. That same month, the health system was honored by the American Hospital Association's *Hospitals & Health Networks* as one of the "100 Most

As the hospital approached its 100th birthday, it had more than fulfilled the mission that its founders envisioned. The entire health system serves as a beacon of light for the sick and the injured. Even more, it serves as a focal point for health. Thanks to its synergistic relationship with the community, Anne Arundel Health System stands poised to face new challenges in the years ahead and to foster a healthy region well into its second century.

S ince I served in the Army Medical Service Corps from 1968 to 1971, I knew I wanted a career in health care.

I feel that what we're doing has a higher purpose. When I walk around the hospital, I'm aware that people are putting their trust in us. I feel particularly fortunate to have spent my career here in Annapolis—the community support has been fantastic, and I'm so proud of the quality of our services, our medical staff and our employees.

And now we have a whole new opportunity with our new hospital. We'll have a facility equal to the quality of care we've been able to deliver, with a healing environment that will enhance that care. It's been a pleasure for me to be a part of the initial dream—from the bare land, to the concept, planning, construction and opening—and to still be here to see it all happen. It has to be a highlight of my career. But I'm not done yet—I continue to look forward to our next phases of development.

At the same time, we all feel sentimental about the old hospital. Almost every room there has a memory for me—my sons were born there; I've had close friends die there, too. It is hard to say goodbye to the old building, but we'll continue to provide services for downtown residents.

No one person is responsible for how far this hospital has come. Collectively, we've recognized the needs of the community and we've met those needs. We've had tremendous community support because we've done what we've said we'd do. We've used openness, flexibility and creativity. We've taken risks. We've looked ahead.

We'll face key challenges in the years ahead. We'll have to continue to make the best use of our financial resources to meet the needs of an aging population. We'll have to keep up with the latest medical developments and meet the challenges of staff shortages. We'll need to continue to attract board members who can look ahead.

I'm very proud of this place—the quality of our services, our staff and our facilities. Most gratifying to me has been the community support we've received. I take it all very personally. You have to, in order to be effective.

Perspective...

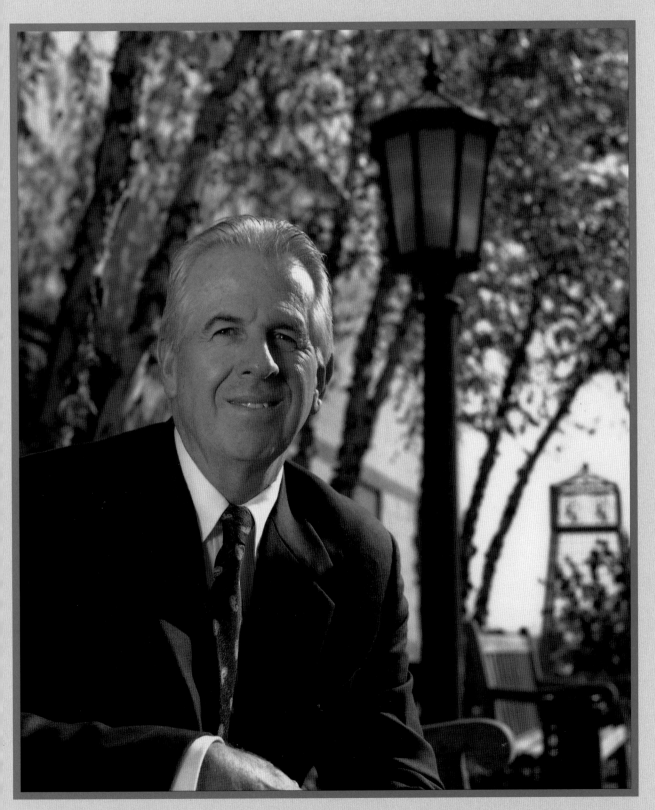

Martin L. "Chip" Doordan

Joined hospital as administrative resident, 1972

AAMC president, 1988

AAHS president, 1994-present

As Anne Arundel Medical Center approached the historic move of its center of operations from downtown Annapolis to Jennifer Road, administrators, physicians, employees and community members alike struggled with two very different emotions. They were visibly excited at the prospect of an all-new Acute Care Pavilion, built to include what they most wanted in a hospital. But at the same time, they were palpably sad about leaving behind their beloved old hospital, where many had said 'hello' and 'good-bye' to loved ones and others had worked for years.

In the weeks leading up to Moving Day— slated for December 2, 2001—there was a groundswell of activity and a growing sense of anticipation. At a black-tie event on November 10 for 1,000 major donors, members of the medical staff and community leaders, chandeliers suspended from the ceiling of a 165' x 60' tent cast a golden glow on guests. Outside, the new hospital's logo was visible

through the tent's clear plastic roof. AAHS president Martin L. "Chip" Doordan honored Hillard Donner, chairman of the "New Century of Caring" capital campaign, and Lisa Hillman, vice president of development and community affairs, thanking them for their role in leading the community to make the new hospital a reality.

At an open house for 1,500 staff members and volunteers on November 11 and another open house for 4,500 community members on November 17, attendees gazed with wonder at the new Acute Care Pavilion. On November 11, a special 24-page section of *The Capital* provided a close-up view of the new hospital to its legions of readers.

During an emotional dedication ceremony on November 13, a bright blue sky framed the new building as a crowd of more than 600 viewed the new hospital through the clear-top tent. Color guards from the Maryland State Police, the Anne Arundel County Fire

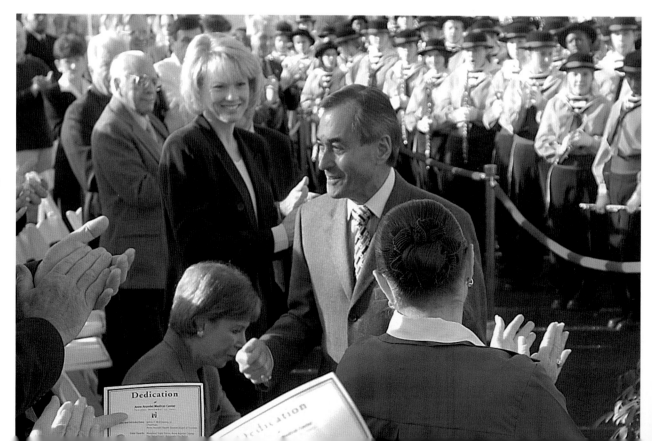

Hillard Donner, chair of the "New Century of Caring" capital campaign and $1 million donor, receives a standing ovation from hundreds of grateful community members at the dedication of the new hospital on November 13, 2001.

A New Hospital, A New Century *2001 - 2002*

Department and the Annapolis Police Department set a patriotic tone for the event. Faye Hunt-Anderson, R.N., a clinical coordinator of AAMC's Outreach Center, thrilled the crowd with a stirring rendition of the National Anthem.

One by one, honored guests—including Lieutenant Governor Kathleen Kennedy Townsend, County Executive Janet Owens and American Hospital Association Richard J. Davidson—voiced their admiration in remarks punctuated by standing ovations. As the Annapolis High School Band and the Weems Creek Nursery School and Kindergarten looked on, officials cut the ribbon and dedicated the new facility to the next generation. Hillard Donner was awarded a standing ovation for his fundraising leadership, and Carl A. "Chuck" Brunetto was acknowledged for his leadership in the development of Medical Park. Carolyn Core, vice president of corporate services, was presented with a collage of images depicting the construction of the new hospital, in honor of her hard work overseeing each detail of the hospital's construction.

"This [new hospital] has special meaning in today's world. How reassuring it is to open a facility that reaffirms life. Can you think of a better birthplace for our second century of caring? If you think we're proud of this place, you're right!"

Martin L. "Chip" Doordan
AAHS President

"This fantastic high-tech facility will enable the medical staff to provide the highest level of care to everyone.

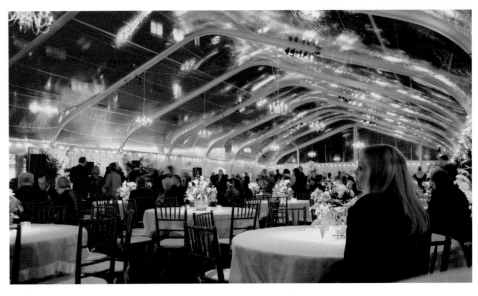

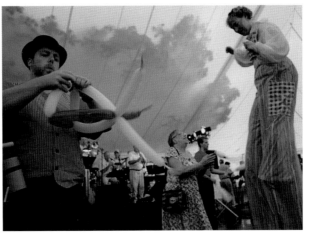

A super-sized tent provided the venue for pre-opening festivities that included a black-tie preview of the new Acute Care Pavilion.

Rain couldn't dampen AAMC's 99th birthday party, which was the last public event held at the downtown hospital. A stilt walker and balloon maker added to the festivities.

No other hospital in this country has this level of sophistication and comfort. We are second to none."

Dr. Michael S. Epstein
President of AAMC Medical Staff

During several trial runs prior to the move, medical staff members and employees rehearsed moving patients and delivering services at the new site. They responded to 22 different patient-care scenarios, so they would have a chance to try out the new facility before real patients arrived. In the weeks preceding the move, employees participated in orientation sessions to familiarize themselves with their new working environment.

The staff prepared for the move for a year, hiring special consultants to help on moving day and during the early days of transition. A 3/4-inch-thick Patient Move Manual detailed each step. On November 20, several departments began moving across town, including microbiology and the askAAMC telehealth service. Through the week of November 26, little bits of most departments also began the gradual trek, transporting supplies and equipment to the new site.

The hospital stopped scheduling elective surgery on November 29, and discharged as many patients as possible prior to the move. The day before the move, some 200 staff members volunteered to put the finishing touches on the new facility. As staffers stocked nursing units and polished the front desk in the lobby, Mr. Doordan and architect Chuck Goodman moved artwork, Chief Operating Officer Sharon Riley unpacked boxes and Vice President of Medical Affairs Dr. Joseph Moser installed patient televisions. Joan Kelly, a 31-year employee, went to every patient room to put stickers on new telephones.

Sunday, December 2, was clear and unseasonably warm. At both facilities, staff members gathered shortly after 5 a.m. to get their marching orders for the day's events. "Today we become part of history," Mr. Doordan told some 200 staff members in the old hospital's cafeteria. "In less than an hour, we open our new hospital. And before the day's end, after 99 years at this site, we close this one. Today is an ending, and a very exciting beginning." At the same time, Sharon Riley delivered a similar message to some 150 staff members at Medical Park.

Their remarks set the tone for the day. Participants alternated between nostalgia for the past and excitement for the future. Mr. Doordan spent the morning traveling between the two universes, bridging both emotions. Alongside much of the time were Sharon Riley, Carolyn Core, Lisa Hillman and Mr. Doordan's son, Sean, who had been born at the old hospital and was on special assign-

Ready, set, go! AAMC staff members assemble on December 2, 2001 at 5 a.m. in the cafeteria of the downtown hospital to go over procedures for moving day.

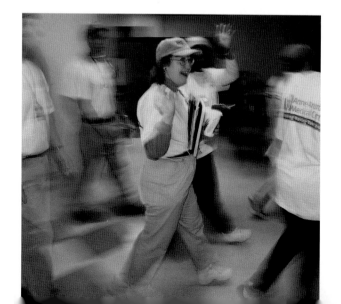

Carolyn Core waves to her coworkers as she heads toward her duty station at the new hospital.

ment there while pursuing a graduate degree in health administration.

At the new facility, emergency department staffers gathered outside the emergency entrance to count down the seconds till 6 a.m., cheering as the hospital and emergency signs lit the pre-dawn sky. "God bless us all," Mr. Doordan said. Then staff members took their posts, as one remarked, "We may get some surprises, so let's be ready."

At the same moment, the old hospital stopped accepting emergency patients, directing them to the new facility. Emergency Department Medical Director Dr. Kenneth Gummerson, Dr. Joseph Halpern and night shift charge nurse William Moore, R.N., stayed behind to continue to care for the patients who remained. That last shift at the old hospital was a highly sought-after shift, and senior staff members were awarded with first pick.

At 6:15 a.m., a fleet of 16 ambulances—from Baltimore, Annapolis and Anne Arundel, Harford, Queen Anne and Baltimore counties—pulled up to the emergency entrance of the downtown hospital to transport 81 patients to the new facility in the hours ahead. As the sun rose over Spa Creek, first out the door at 6:35 a.m. was Frank Woods, an 80-year-old war hero from Dover, Delaware. Simultaneously, a new banner was unfurled outside the entrance, announcing, "This facility is closed." Staff members lined the driveway to wave goodbye to departing patients.

Across town, the first emergency department patient, Ines Ray, arrived by ambulance at 6:20 a.m. with a broken hip. Another patient mistakenly came to the old emergency department at about 6:15 a.m., and was redirected to the new hospital.

At the new hospital's main entrance, the first ambulance pulled up at 6:47 a.m., carrying Mr. Woods. Mr. Doordan and other senior staff members were out front to greet him, bestowing a gift of *Annapolis: A Portrait,* a handsome photographic essay by Roger Miller, and a commemorative AAMC t-shirt. Staff members smiled and clapped. "We're open for business," remarked Lucy Peacock, a customer information assistant at the front desk.

Shortly after 8 a.m., Auxiliary members began reporting to duty. Irma Myers and Len Klaver went to work in the emergency department. Jean Giden took her place behind the front desk in the lobby. Maryalice Bassford also was on hand.

As the day wore on, the intricate plan to ensure a seamless continuum of care throughout the move picked up pace. At the old hospital, move commander Beth Evins, vice president of quality improvement services, and Patricia Travis, director of medical-surgical services, manned the control desk to monitor departing patients. Six teams were responsible for moving different departments.

Each patient left the hospital surrounded by paramedics and nursing staff. The caring was evident as nurses tucked blankets around an unconscious young man, in an effort to ease his ambulance ride.

A custom-designed software program tracked each step of the patient move. As patients left the old facility, their names appeared in green on computer monitors at the old and new hospitals, along with their admitting physician's name and their new bed assignment. Then when patients arrived, the color changed to red to indicate their arrival. In this

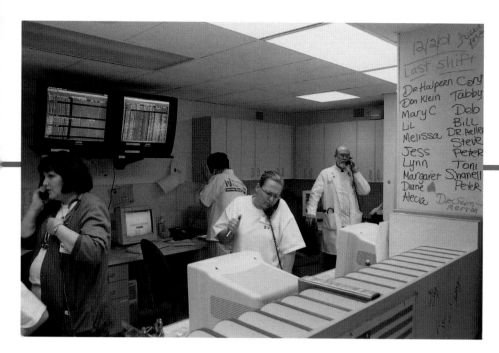

The handwritten note on the whiteboard reads:
12/2/01
Last shift
Dr Halpeen Cory
Don Klein Tabby
Mary C Dob
Lil Bill
Melissa Dr. Aeller
  Steve
Jess Peter
Lynn Toni
Margaret Shanell
Diane Peter
Alecia Dr. Siem
  Merton

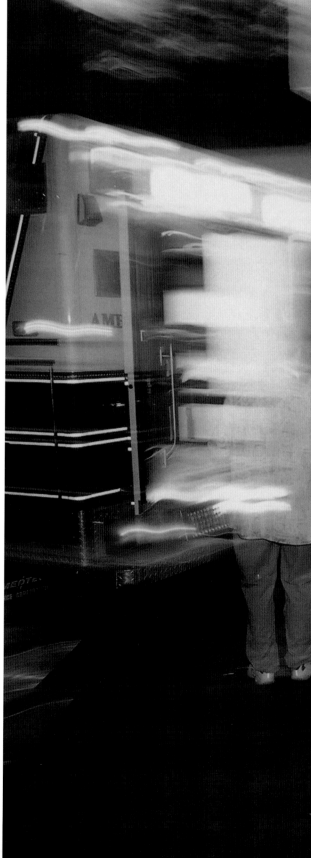

The last shift at the downtown emergency department is still on the job at 7 a.m. as they cleared the remaining patients from their area. On the column above the main desk, they commemorated the "Last Shift" of workers at the old hospital.

The entrance to the downtown hospital (right) is a beehive of activity on Moving Day. Sixteen ambulances from the surrounding area lent a hand moving patients to the Medical Park campus.

way, all patients were tracked—and, more importantly, cared for—each step of the way.

Across town at the new hospital, Vickie Diamond, clinical administrator of medical services; and Sue Patton, clinical director of surgical services, tracked the arriving patients. They made certain that patients were transferred to the appropriate beds. Dr. Moser served as troubleshooter, keeping a close watch on the proceedings throughout the day.

The clinical staff determined the sequence in which patients were moved. Each unit took turns transferring patients to distribute the workload evenly in the new facility, usually sending the sickest patients first. Downtown hospital nurses briefed transport nurses on each patient's condition. Then the transport nurse handed off care to a nurse on the receiving end at the new hospital. County and city police directed traffic along the ambulance route to facilitate the move.

At 8:15 a.m., Barbara Pease became the first surgical patient. Dr. David Weintritt performed a 45-minute laparoscopic appendectomy on Mrs. Pease, who had registered at the old emergency department the night before and been one of the first patients to be transferred to the new facility. Dr. Marshall K. Steele III, medical director of surgical services, was on hand through the morning to make sure things went smoothly.

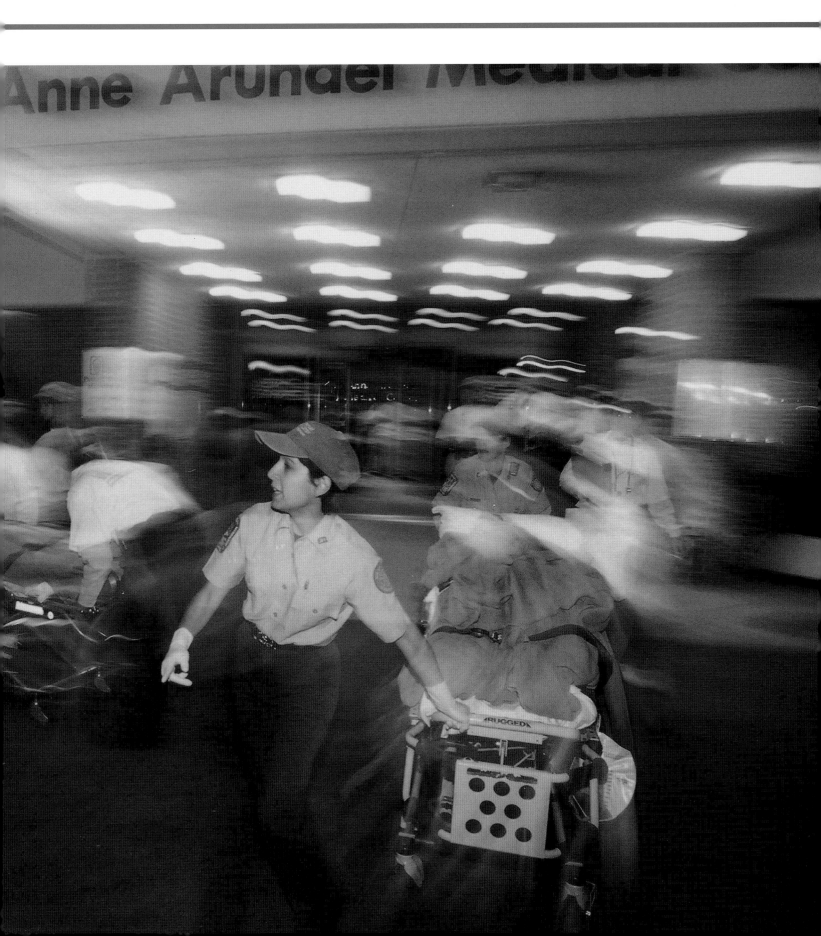

THE FIRST INPATIENT TRANSFER

On Friday, November 30, Jack R. Woods of Dover, Delaware stopped for lunch in Annapolis on his way to Baltimore-Washington International Airport. A Pearl Harbor survivor, he was on his way to Honolulu to commemorate the 60th anniversary of the attack. Instead, the 80-year-old retired public works director woke up at the old Anne Arundel Medical Center, after fainting at a local restaurant.

Two days later, he was the first patient to be transferred from the old hospital to the new Acute Care Pavilion at Medical Park. He left to applause at 6:35 a.m. and arrived to still more applause at 6:47. "People have been absolutely tremendous," he says. "I feel like I'm Clark Gable. I think the new hospital is lovely. I was on the hospital board in Dover for seven years, so I know what a good hospital is."

Despite the excitement, his care proceeded without interruption, under the watchful eye of Dr. Douglas S. Mitchell, a hospitalist. Nurses checked on him frequently and he was ushered downstairs for an MRI exam within hours of the new hospital's opening.

THE FIRST SURGERY PATIENT

Barbara Pease, 27, a kindergarten teacher at Mayo Elementary School, had experienced abdominal pain before, but this was different. Her husband, Gordon, suspected appendicitis and urged her to go the emergency room. The two Edgewater residents entered the downtown hospital's emergency department on Saturday, December 1, at 10:30 p.m. A CAT scan proved Gordon right.

At 4:30 a.m. on Sunday, she was admitted to the downtown hospital and promptly put on the surgery schedule at the new hospital, which would open in less than two hours. She was one of the first patients transferred to Medical Park by ambulance, arriving about 7 a.m. She went directly to the second floor to be prepared for surgery.

Down the hall, Dr. David Weintritt, the newest surgeon on the medical staff, assembled his team and prepared to perform the new hospital's first operation. The laparoscopic appendectomy started at 8:15 a.m. and lasted just 45 minutes. "These operating rooms are bigger and more user-friendly," Dr. Weintritt noted. "Everything went beautifully." Another plus was the portable overhead monitor that allowed him a better view of the patient's abdomen.

"I've never been a patient in a hospital before," Mrs. Pease said, as she rested in her private hospital room afterwards. "Everyone's been so friendly." Her husband added, "This is an amazing hospital."

THE FIRST EMERGENCY PATIENT

The first ambulance pulled up to the new Acute Care Pavilion's ambulance entrance at 6:20 a.m. on Sunday, December 2, just 20 minutes after the hospital opened for business. Inside the ambulance was 71-year-old Ines Ray, who had fallen at her Cape St. Claire home the night before.

The emergency department staff sprang into action. An X-ray showed that Mrs. Ray had a broken hip. The digital image showed up immediately on the physician's computer monitor, appearing simultaneously on the radiologist's screen to confirm the diagnosis. "This new technology is amazing," agreed Dr. C. Michael Remoll and Dr. Melissa Mikami, emergency department physicians. "It really speeds up care."

The First Patients...

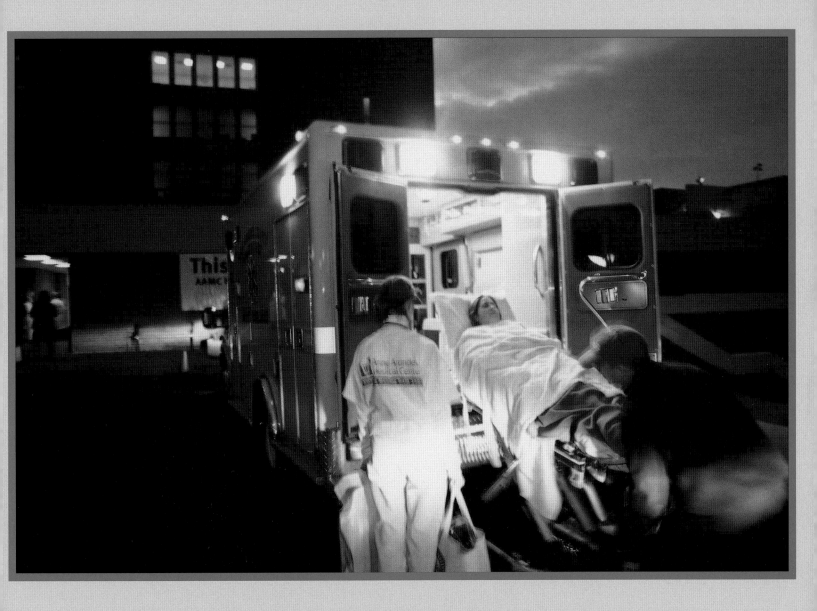

"This is absolutely wonderful," said Sharon Jernigan, Mrs. Ray's daughter. "It's very organized for the first day." Like many local residents, Mrs. Jernigan was no stranger to Anne Arundel Medical Center—as a child she was a patient in the old part of the hospital, her children were born at the downtown hospital, and her granddaughter was one of the first babies born at the Clatanoff Pavilion. Further, her family's concrete pumping business par-

ticipated in the construction of the new facility.

Mrs. Ray had hip repair surgery the next day, performed by Dr. Christina M. Morganti. She then spent her 72nd birthday on December 4 in a private room, enjoying a birthday cake prepared in the cafeteria. "This room is very nice," she said, "and they've treated me well." Her daughter agreed, saying, "I give it a thumbs up, and I mean a real thumbs up!"

Barbara Pease, the first surgery patient at the new Acute Care Pavilion, is placed in an ambulance at dawn at the downtown facility for the trip to the new hospital.

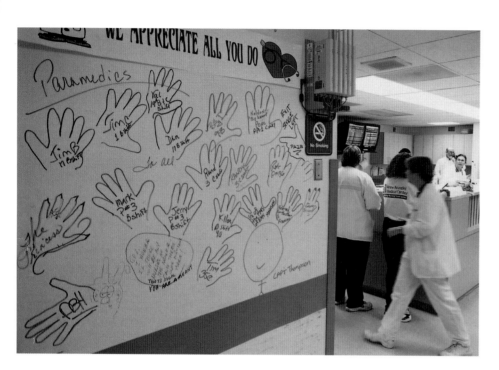

At the new hospital, the people who had played such an important role in its construction were on hand through the morning. Architect Chuck Goodman stood by, watching his design come to life. Similarly, Randy Thomas, construction manager for J. Vinton Schafer & Sons, Inc., was present, available to solve problems, should any arise. None did. Workers were seen behind the scenes, ready to help staff members with minor problems. Carolyn Core; Dennis Curl, vice president of property development; and Charles "Charlie" Steele, Clerk of the Works, were everywhere, overseeing their final product.

The feeling of excitement was pervasive throughout the new hospital. But on the floors, the care was reassuringly routine. Just an hour after opening, nurses were busy tending to patients and physicians made rounds while patients rested comfortably in their private rooms. Most noticeable was the quiet that prevailed, made possible by the thorough preparation, carpeted hallways and silent communication systems. "The patients are getting in and getting settled," said Myra Landmesser, R.N., director of nursing in the critical care unit. The technology performed flawlessly.

The new emergency department filled quickly. Patients sat quietly in the spacious new waiting room, remarking on the comfort of the new facility. A television at one end played softly. In the pediatric waiting room, a young mother with a sick child lying across her lap, remarked, "I was dreading coming to the emergency room, but this is wonderful. It's been a very pleasant experience." Outside, a father and daughter walked through the Healing Garden.

Doctors and nurses, too, were thrilled with the space, the efficiency, the quiet and the new technology. "Everything has gone very smoothly," said James Dyson, R.N., nursing supervisor for the emergency department. "The process has changed, so we've had to be flexible. But that's what we're good at."

Downtown, the old hospital rapidly emptied. Inpatients left by ambulance in an orderly procession. By 7:20 a.m., the emergency department had just nine patients. As patients were discharged, physicians and staff members signed the walls with colorful tracings of hands, signatures and even some personal remembrances from nurses who'd met their husbands there.

The last emergency patient left before 11:30 a.m. "It's been very orderly," said Dr. Joseph Halpern, a 14-year veteran. "It's almost anticlimactic now." But the feeling of nostalgia was everywhere. As the emergency department emptied, staff members—along with Mr. Doordan

—congregated near the nurses' desk to reminisce about their years there. "My father died in this emergency room," Dr. Gummerson remembered.

Upstairs, care continued as usual, even as the floors emptied of patients. Dr. Stanley P. Watkins, Jr., medical director of oncology services, made his sixth-floor rounds for the last time, checking in on his patients and moving boxes. Dr. Vernon Croft, department chairman of medicine, helped out, too.

Precisely at 1:10 p.m., the last inpatient left the downtown hospital. The lobby clock was stopped to commemorate the moment. Mr. Doordan, Board Chairman James McEneaney, Jr. and others escorted the last patient, Sandra McCarthy, from her room on A6, as she was wheeled out to staff members' applause. "I'm a little nostalgic, but I'm so excited," Mr. McEneaney remarked. Nurses watched with tears in their eyes, among them long-time nurse Catherine Copertino, clinical administrator of oncology.

The A3 staff celebrates the closing of their area by participating in a series of high (and low) fives with fellow employees.

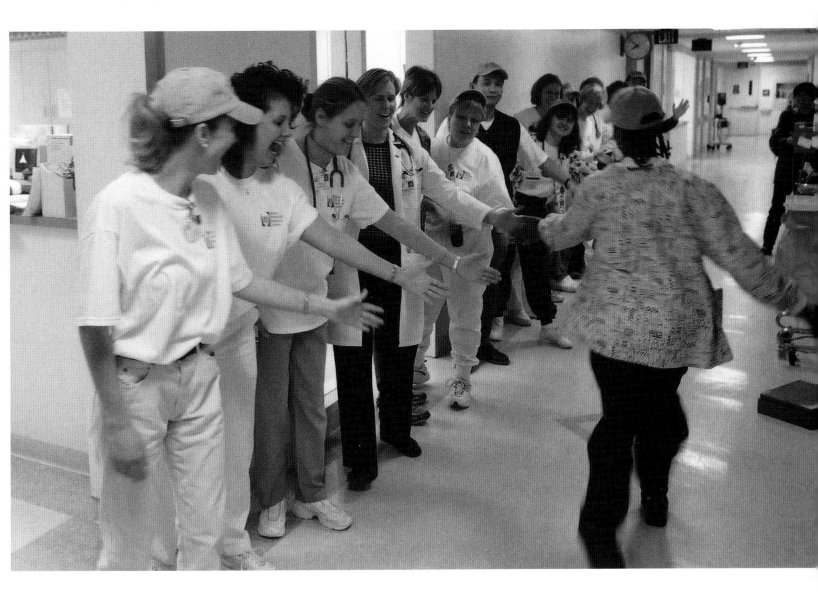

As the Annapolis City ambulance pulled away accompanied by a three-car police escort, Mr. Doordan declared, "This building is now closed to patient care." Throughout the morning, neighbors walked by to watch the goings-on and staff members visited for the last time. Physicians—including Dr. Elizabeth Maxwell-Schmidt, associate chief of emergency services—showed up with their children to observe the historic transition.

"This has been A+ planning," said Sedonna Brown, R.N., as she watched the last patient leave the downtown hospital's driveway. "This is a new era for Annapolis," added Barbara Emert, R.N. Fittingly, the sun chose that time to shine brightly for the first time that day.

The last patient arrived at the new hospital shortly after 1:15 p.m. to cheers and waves. Mrs. McCarthy was promptly wheeled upstairs. When all was said and done, the biggest surprise was that there were no surprises during the move. Mr. Doordan shook his head in wonder at the ease of the move. "They're [the staff] a class act, aren't they?" he remarked. "The move went as well as we planned, and even better than we thought," Beth Evins added.

Inside the old hospital, various pieces of equipment remained, some to be moved and some to be discarded. Many workers had signed walls throughout the hospital. On A6 the walls read, "Hospital Closed. Gone Fishin'," "So many of us got our wings here," and "Thank you for being there for [our family]. My mom has been one of the many who have been touched by you all."

Some staff members stayed on to help close the building, with the engineering department scheduled as the last to leave in late December. A banner draped the building, announcing, "This facility is closed. Anne Arundel Medical Center has moved to 2001 Medical Parkway." The windows were boarded up as the New Year began, and Madison Homes began preparations to convert the property into a residential development.

In its first 24 hours of operation, the new Acute Care Pavilion admitted 24 new patients and treated 146 patients in the emergency department. By the middle of the week, the hospital was fully operational. Despite a high level of activity throughout, serenity prevailed. The operating and procedure rooms were working at full tilt, the emergency department was seeing an increased number of patients, and most beds were filled. With the new hospital's early success, the staff was already looking forward to opening the sixth floor in January.

Doctors marveled at the beauty and technology in the new facility. Nurses remarked on how much more efficient the new setup was. Patients and families were most pleased of all. "Patients report that they're sleeping better and having less pain," Beth Evins said. "And the space is more efficient, so nurses are able to focus their efforts on spending time with and educating their patients. It's a win-win for everyone."

Elsewhere on the Medical Park campus, business continued as usual throughout the week. Babies were born in the Clatanoff Pavilion and outpatient surgeries took place at the Edwards Pavilion. Similarly, patients visited their doctors' offices at the Wayson and Sajak Pavilions, and sought cancer care in the Donner Pavilion. Administrators moved into their new offices in the Sajak Pavilion, already planning for the years ahead.

"The new hospital is a major milestone for Anne Arundel Health System. This is a dynamic, growing organization and we are committed to keeping pace with our community's needs, as well as providing the quality of health care this community deserves."

Sharon Riley
Chief Operating Officer
Anne Arundel Health System

"The move's success reflects the professionalism and careful attention to detail that we have grown accustomed to....When it comes to hospital care, this region is in good hands."

Editorial in *The Capital*
December 5, 2001

At the entrance to the new emergency department at Medical Park, employees cheer as the new sign lights promptly at 6 a.m. and they are officially "open for business."

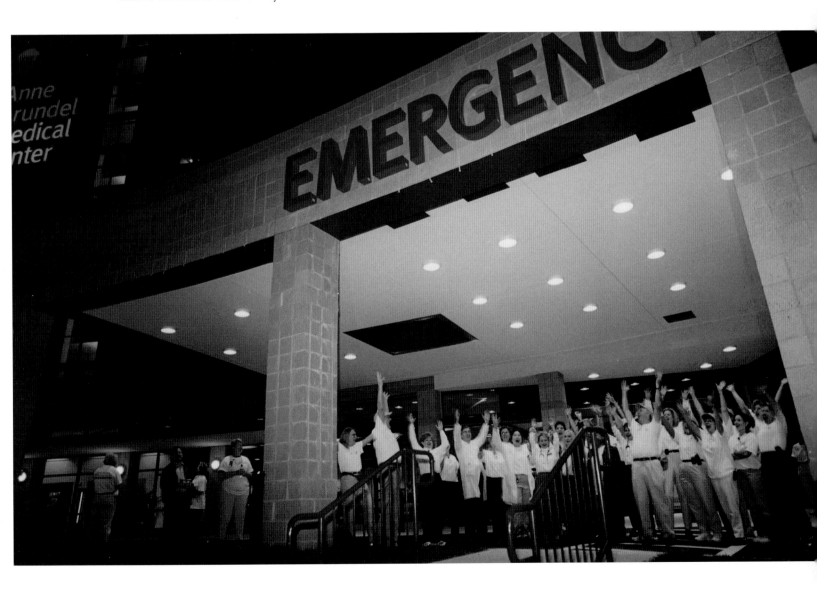

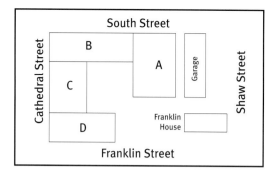

Locations given below refer to designations of the downtown hospital buildings. A is the South Building or tower, B is the Baldwin Building, C is the 1928 annex and D is the Franklin Street building, built in 1910.

1902, February 17: Annapolis Emergency Hospital Association incorporated by 10 women and Mayor Charles A. Dubois.

1902, May 31: Property of Edwin A. Seidewitz on Franklin and Cathedral streets purchased for the hospital.

1902, July 18: Annapolis Emergency Hospital admitted its first patient.

1909: Construction began on Franklin Street building.

1910, December: New hospital on Franklin Street opened; dedication held on December 5, 1910.

1911, February: Emergency Hospital Training School for Nurses opened.

1913, December 1: Ida Rose White was the first graduate of the nursing school.

1915: First maternity ward established by Dr. Frances E. Weitzman and Nurse Margaret Wohlgemuth.

1918: Hospital association purchased additional land on Franklin Street.

1919: First radiology department opened with one X-ray machine.

1920: Nurses' Home on Franklin Street completed.

1922: First clinical laboratory established.

1925: Dietitian added to hospital staff.

1927, December 16: Hospital gutted by fire.

1928, March 9: Cornerstone laid for the annex on Cathedral Street.

1928, September: Renovated main building reopened for use after fire.

1930, November 14: Annex on Cathedral Street opened.

1934: The hospital received its first accreditation from the American College of Surgeons.

1935: Training School for Nurses closed.

1944: Hospital Auxiliary founded.

1944: Loran S. Messick hired as administrator of the hospital.

1945: Men elected to the Board of Managers for the first time since 1902. John B. Rich named board president.

1947, January: Sherrill S. Adams appointed administrator.

1948: Hospital received title to the land under D building from the state.

1949, November: Hospital's name changed to Anne Arundel General Hospital.

1951: John B. Rich Building constructed as medical annex (later became the pediatric unit and eventually demolished to make way for the A building).

1952: Dr. Frank M. Shipley named chief of medicine, the first local chief of service.

1952: Clothes Box opened by the hospital Auxiliary.

1952: Auxiliary offered rental radio service to patients.

1952: Dr. Manning W. Alden hired as full-time pathologist.

1952, August: Anne Arundel General Hospital was one of first hospitals in Maryland to require routine chest X-rays of patients.

1952, November: Construction begun on Summerfield Baldwin, Jr. Memorial Wing.

1953, June: School for practical nurses opened.

1953: Anesthesia service established with physician-anesthesiologist.

1954: Charles B. Lynch Memorial Library established.

1954: Dr. Raymond L. Richardson joined the staff as the hospital's first black physician of the modern period.

1955: Black maternity patients admitted to the hospital.

1955, May 12: Summerfield Baldwin, Jr. Memorial Wing (B) dedicated.

1956: Radioisotopes first used in diagnostic procedures.

1958, February: Lyman C. Whittaker hired as hospital's first professional administrator.

1958, July: The hospital received full accreditation from the Joint Commission on the Accreditation of Hospitals.

1959: Carl A. Brunetto joined the hospital as assistant administrator.

Chronology

1959: Hospital contracted with outside company for food service.

1960: Hospital pharmacy established.

1961: Rental television service by the Auxiliary began.

1966: James R. Martin Coronary Care Unit established.

1966: The first Pink Lady Ball, sponsored by the hospital Auxiliary, held.

1967: Auxiliary began closed circuit broadcasting on the hospital's own television channel.

1967: Intensive care unit established.

1968: Special care unit established.

1969, November 22: South, or A, Building dedicated.

1971: Physical therapy service established.

1971: Pulmonary function service established.

1972: Martin L. Doordan began his association with Anne Arundel General Hospital.

1972: Hospital food service again made an in-house operation.

1973: Nuclear medicine service established.

1974: Electroencephalography service established.

1976, June: New Cathedral Street wing opened with expanded emergency services department.

1976: CAT scanner in operation at the hospital.

1977: First total hip replacement, by Dr. Robert Ellis.

1977: Psychiatric service established.

1978, April 25: Name of hospital association changed to Anne Arundel General Hospital, Inc.

1978, July: Psychiatric unit opened on the sixth floor of A building.

1979, September: Parking garage opened.

1979: Lyman C. Whittaker retired and Carl A. Brunetto became administrator.

1980: First total knee replacement, by Dr. Stephen Faust.

1981: Hospital hospice program established.

1983: Outpatient IV therapy inaugurated.

1983: Engineering department established.

1983: Anne Arundel General Hospital Foundation incorporated.

1983: First percutaneous kidney stone surgery performed.

1984: First revascularization procedure, by Drs. David Lowe, C. William Strawberry, D. Paul Buhrer.

1984: Home health program began.

1984: The hospital association purchased 104 acres of land on Jennifer Road.

1985: On-line linkage established between the hospital library and the National Library of Medicine.

1985: Anne Arundel Diagnostics centers opened in Annapolis and Arnold.

1985: Podiatry service established.

1986: Department of pastoral care opened with hospital's first chaplain, Rev. Lee Waltz.

1986: First hospital-based MRI unit opened on Jennifer Road.

1986, September: Anne Arundel Diagnostics opened radiology center at Crofton.

1987: Full-time, in-house pediatric coverage established under contract with Drs. Dwight Fortier and Robert Graw.

1987, November: Construction begun on Medical Park buildings.

1988, March: Hospital association's name changed to Anne Arundel General Health Care Systems, Inc.

1988, December: Kent Island radiology clinic opened.

1989: Hospital's name changed to Anne Arundel Medical Center.

1989: Medical Park oncology, outpatient surgery and health education centers opened.

1990: Pathways treatment center planned with county and state agencies.

1991, March: First retina surgery, by Dr. David R. Watt.

1991, September: Association bylaws changed to enable Board of Trustees to elect new board members.

1992, July: Hospital celebrates 90th birthday.

1992, October: Pathways opens.

1993, February: Cardiac cath lab opens.

1993, August: Construction of Phase II Medical Park begins.

CHRONOLOGY (CONTINUED)

1994, February: Auxiliary celebrates 50th birthday.

1994: Outreach Clinic at Lighthouse Shelter opens.

1994: Anne Arundel Diagnostics in Kent Island opens.

1994, June: AAGHCS and AAMC boards merge; Carl Brunetto becomes president emeritus and Martin Doordan becomes president and CEO of AAHS; name changed to AAHS.

1995, September: Clatanoff and Medical Office pavilions open.

1995: Breast Center established.

1996: Center for Joint Replacement opens.

1996, March: Chuck Brunetto retires.

1996: ASK-A-NURSE Program established.

1996, Oct. 31: Board endorses concept of consolidation of inpatient services at Medical Park.

1997, May: Third floor of Clatanoff Pavilion opens.

1997: AAHS web site established.

1997, Fall: Shipley's Choice Medical Park opens.

1997: Diabetes Resource Center established.

1997, October: New plans for hospital unveiled.

1998: Spine Center and Sleep Disorders Center established.

1998: Level III+ designation awarded to NICU at Clatanoff Pavilion.

1998: Annapolis Outreach Center opens.

1998: AAMC enters into agreement with Nighttime Pediatrics.

1998: AAMC wins Mercury Award as #1 hospital overall in Baltimore region.

1998, Dec. 16: Groundbreaking for new hospital.

1999: Maternal/Fetal Medicine Program established.

1999: AAMC named one of nation's Top 100 Hospitals for Orthopedics by HCIA.

1999, June: Groundbreaking for West Campus.

1999, September: Madison Homes selected as developer for downtown hospital site.

1999: AAHS transfers home health and hospice service to MedStar Health.

2000: Web site expanded to include physician referral and HealthGate information network.

2000, July: AAMC named by *U.S. News & World Report*'s America's 50 Best Hospitals for gynecology and respiratory disorders.

2000, Jan.1: New Year dawns with no computer glitches!

2000, April: AAMC signs agreement with Kaiser Permanente as regional referral center.

2000, Apr. 20: Topping off of new hospital.

2000: Vascular Institute and Maryland Neurological Institute established.

2000, July: AAMC Outreach Center opens in Stanton Community Center.

2001, February: AAMC Health Services— *Bowie* opens.

2001, March: Sajak Pavilion opens with new Breast Center as centerpiece.

2001: AAMC signs agreement with Children's National Medical Center for provision of pediatric hospitalist services.

2001: AAHS leases space at Village at Waugh Chapel to establish medical offices, diagnostics and urgent care.

2001, July 18: 99th birthday party held on grounds of downtown hospital.

2001, July: AAHS named to "100 Most Wired Hospitals and Health Care Systems" list by *Hospitals & Health Networks*.

2001, Nov. 13: Dedication ceremony for Acute Care Pavilion.

2001, Dec. 2: AAMC leaves downtown hospital and moves all services to Medical Park.

2002, Jan. 3: Acute Care Pavilion's sixth floor opens.

2002, January: Wound Care Center opens.

Statistics

A REPRESENTATIVE SAMPLING OF STATISTICS DECADE BY DECADE OVER THE HOSPITAL'S 100 YEARS

	1904*	1911	1920	1931	1941	1951	1961	1971	1981	1991	2001
Admissions	50	300	676	1,347	2,359	4,042	9,712	10,268	13,432	15,965	19,993
ER visits		2,119	1,349	1,897	2,842	4,367	15,480	28,465	35,711	39,601	55,463
Births			106	148	366	719	1,529	1,416	2,083	2,917	4,399
Deaths	6	22	27	58	77	94	219				
Surgical procedures	8	422	258	644	919	1,345	3,715	5,560	8,830	16,819	18,688
Laboratory tests					408	31,107	113,569			310,274 (1990)	597,168
X-rays			500	1,406	1,238	3,265	20,267		46,911	90,346 (1990)	109,666
Average stay (days)			12.25	13	c. 7	6	6.52		6.54	5.06	3.23
Budget (Operating)	$4,112	$11,404		$85,614		$334,745	$2,043,818		$25,830,937	$88,919,000	$173,321,000
Operating income vs. expenses	17% gain			2% loss		3.9% loss	2.5% gain		1.4% loss	3% gain	4.6% gain
Patient beds	11	30	42	100		85	200	c. 249	288	303	244
Anne Arundel County Population	1900: 39,620	1910: 39,553	1920: 43,408	1930: 55,167	1940: 68,375	1950: 117,392	1960: 206,634	1970: 298,042	1980: 370,775	1990: 427,239	2000: 489,656

Note: These figures were taken from the reports of the chief of the medical staff or the treasurer for the years shown. Figures for all categories for all years were not available, and some were interpolated. 1904 is the first full year of operation for which statistics were given. Population figures for Anne Arundel County were supplied by the Annapolis Office of Planning and Zoning.

Anne Arundel Health System, Inc.

Anne Arundel Medical Center
    Anne Arundel Diagnostics
    Pathways

Anne Arundel Medical Center Foundation

Anne Arundel Real Estate Holding Company
    Pavilion Park

Anne Arundel Health Care Enterprises

APPRECIATION

Anne Arundel Medical Center wishes to acknowledge all the individuals who have helped to advance health care in the community during this institution's first 100 years. Only a small number of those names could be listed here. Others are cherished in the memories of those who knew them. AAMC thanks them all.

Appendix

Jessie K. Garrison (Mrs. David M.) 1916–1919
Mary I. Gassaway (Mrs. L. Dorsey) 1908–1918
Ellen T. Gearing (Mrs Henry C.) 1902–1903
F. Elmer Gelhaus 1969–1977
Nancy Gideon (Mrs. William G.) 1963–1965
Sadie R. Gilden (Mrs. Meyer W.) 1949–1953
Calvin W. Gray 1990–1997
Frances B. Green (Mrs. Nicholas H.) 1901–1919
Mrs. Angelo Hall 1912–1917
Jimmy R. Hammond 1980–
Charlotte R. Harbold (Mrs. Robert P.) 1938–1939
J. Fred Hawkins, Jr., M.D. 1962
John L. Hedeman, M.D. 1960–1961
Virginia T. Heise (Mrs. Edward C.) 1920–1923
Margaret Heller 1922–1928
Robert E. Henel, Jr. 1999-
Edward M. Herrmann 1963–1966
Robertson C. Hesse 1977–1980
Noah A. Hillman 1946–1952
Beatrice Hiltabidle (Mrs. Walter) 1949–1950
Richard I. Hochman, M.D. 1985–1987
Mrs. C. Addison Hodges 1950–1951
Miriam I. Holladay (Mrs. W. Meade) 1911–1919
H. Logan Holtgrewe, M.D. 1973–1975, 1975–1981
Donald E. Hood 1973–1976
Margaret G. Hood (Mrs. Donald E.) 1971–1972,
    1976–1982
John K. Hopkins 1985–2002
Theodore G. Hoster 1957–1970, #1965
Elizabeth H. Iliff, M.D. 1958–1961
Elmer M. Jackson, Jr. 1961–1963, #1961
Dorothy O. Jacobs (Mrs. Harry A.) 1943–1946
Jane H. Jacobsen (Mrs. Jacob) 1991–1994
Anne Burton Jeffers (Mme. Alexandre
Daussoigne–Mehul) 1904–1907
*Jeanette C. Joachim (Mrs. William F.) 1941–1944,
    1951–1952*
Rev. Dr. Robert L. Jones 1945–1948
J. Reaney Kelly 1956–1958
Elsie M. Kemp (Mrs. W. Thomas) 1932–1941
Mrs. Paul J. Kiefer 1923–1942
George M. King 1982–1986
Elizabeth M. Kingsley, M.D. 1999-
Florence B. Kurdle 1992-1999
Jack Kushner, M.D. 1978–1981
Elizabeth H. Labrot (Mrs. Sylvester W.) 1923–1926
Marguerite L. Labrot (Mrs. William H.) 1944–1950
Mrs. Arthur Langfield 1920–1923

Michael J. LaPenta, M.D. 1996-2000
Jerome LaPides 1964–1975
Mrs. Frank H. Lash 1932–1935
Elizabeth F. Lee (Mrs. C. Carroll) 1965–1971
Jon B. Lowe, M.D. 1991–
Charles B. Lynch 1949–1958, #1955
Rev. Dr. James F. Madison 1962–1965
Ray W. Marriner 1975–1979
M. Lee Marston 1996-
*Phoebe E. Martin (Mrs. John W.) 1902–1916**
Cynthia McBride 1999-
Albert H. McCarthy 1946–1952
Catharine C. McComas (Mrs. Joseph P.) 1902–1903*
Mary C. McCormick (Mrs. Howard C.) 1947–1958
Michael V. McCutchan 1978–1995
James F. McEneaney, Jr. 1994-
David S. McHold, M.D. 1983–1985
Mary E. McMakin (Mrs. J. F.) 1905–1919
Daniel W. McNew 1982–2000
Walter C. McNiel 1957–1960
*Hon. William J. McWilliams 1951–1965
    (life member, 1963)*
Jean Meehla (Mrs. John B.) 1976–1978
John B. Melvin 1961–1990, #1967
Augusta B. Melvin (Mrs. Ridgely P.) 1924–1925
Helen M. Merriam (Mrs. George A.) 1903–1904
Lulu O. Merrill (Mrs. George E.) 1903–1910
Amelia E. Miller (Mrs. George A.) 1903–1905
Norman A. Miller, Jr. 1972–1975
Selda V. Miller (Mrs. Philip) 1925–1943, 1944–1946
Elizabeth Mitchell (Mrs. Carleton) 1950–1957
Thomas G. Moore 1986–1989
Mary S. Moreland (Mrs. Russell) 1952–1956
Louise Morris (Mrs. Karlton F.) 1973–1974
Rear Adm. (Ret.) Robert M. Morris 1957–1960
Joseph D. Moser, M.D. 1994-1996
April Moses 1993-2001
Elizabeth D. Moss (Mrs. George Abram) 1919–1945
Virginia Mullan 1905–1907
Edward F. Mullen 1983–1989
Lyda J. Munroe (Mrs. Walter C.) 1938–1943
Margaret H. Munroe (Mrs. Frank A.)1907–1911
E. Churchill Murray 1946–1952
Elizabeth M. Murray (Mrs. James D.) 1903–1906
Isabel W. Murray (Mrs. Henry M.) 1958–1964
Irma Myers (Mrs. Benjamin T.) 1967–1969
James L. Myers 2001-
Robert R. Neal 1995-1999

Barbara Niedringhaus (Mrs. John M.) 1951–1958
Francis L. Noel 1974–1977
Harold V. Nutt 1964–1975
Donna M. Olfson (Mrs. James O.) 1980–1986
James O. Olfson 1972–1978
Barber C. Palmer, M.D. 1963–1965
Mrs. Henry M. Paul 1910–1912
Robert C. Paxson, Jr. 1986–1996
Richard N. Peeler, M.D. 1969–1971
James L. Pierce 2001-
Lydia H. Poore (Mrs. Arthur L.) 1942–1945
Mary M. Proskey (Mrs. Alexander S.) 1919–1938
J. Oliver Purvis, M.D. 1945
May V. Quenstedt (Mrs. Walter E.) 1933–1937
David T. Raisen 1954–1958
Kate W. Randall 1903–1922
Barbara Ray 1999-2001
Allen J. Reiter 1959–1965
Pauline W. Remey 1957+
John B. Rich 1945–1965 #1951 (life member, 1958)
Robert L. Rich 1966–1973, #1966
Geneva F. Richards (Mrs. Charles L.) 1983–1985, 1985–1991
William H. Richardson 1951–1954
Sherman S. Robinson, M.D. 1972
Richard D. Rooney 1994-
Rabbi Morris D. Rosenblatt 1958–1961
Patricia Rutemiller 1996-1998
H. Erle Schafer 1972–1974+
Charles L. Schelberg 1972–1975
Ruth Schnell (Mrs. John) 1974–1976
George W. Settle, M.D. 1975–1977
Geraldine Settle (Mrs. George W.) 1978–1980
Bennett H. Shaver 1986–
E. Roy Shawn 1979–1981
Bernadine Sheehan (Mrs. Joseph) 1958–1960
Frank M. Shipley, M.D. 1958
Sidney T. Shores 1974–1984
Joseph N. Shumate 1962–1965
Amelia H. Smith (Mrs. Rudolph M. J.) 1939–1943
Anna Smith (Mrs. Albert A., Jr.) 1981–1983
Donald R. Smith 1964–1978
Malcolm B. Smith 1970–1980, #1976
Martha A. Smith, Ph.D. 2000-
William J. Sneeringer 1953–1960
Jane R. Snider, Ed.D. 1996-2000

Regina Stansbury 1994-1996
Anna B. Steele (Mrs. Nevett) 1903–1904
Charles H. Steele 1980–1986
Claudia M. Stevens (Mrs. William O.) 1920–1924
Ann Stockett 1976–1978+
Esther S. Stone (Mrs. Raymond) 1919–1922
Thomas H. Stone 1948–1951
Louis M. Strauss 1953–1957
Ruth W. Styer (Mrs. Charles A.) 1922–1925
John M. Suit II 1990–2001
Florence N. Tardy (Mrs. Walter B.) 1928–1934
Maj. Gen. J. Francis Taylor, Jr. 1975–1982
Carl A. TenHoopen 1986–1996
Carl J. Tenner 1981–1985, 1991–
Mrs. Terry Thompson 1933–1934?
Julia M. Tisdale (Mrs. Ryland D.) 1912–1935
Mrs. Burnett F. Treat 1944–1947
Patricia Troy 1995-
John Trumpy, Jr. 1960–1966
Alice T. Turner (Mrs. George J.) 1922–1942
George W. Velenovsky 1970–1976
Peter F. Verkouw, M.D. 1980–1982
Evelyn Wainwright (Mrs. Richard) 1902*
Sherburne B. Walker 1958–1991 #1971 (life member, 1978)
David H. Wallace 1952–1956
Katherine Walton 1902–1905*
Emma N. Warfield (Mrs. Edwin) 1904–1907
Dr. Stanley P. Watkins, Jr. 1976–1982
Margaret T. Weems (Mrs. Philip V. H.) 1933–1940
McLean S. Welch 1956–1970, #1962 (life member, 1969)
Robert S. G. Welch, M.D. 1947–1949, 1954–1956
Florine M. Werntz (Mrs. C. Garner) 1943–1946
Elizabeth W. Westcott (Mrs. Allan F.) 1935–1941
Chancy F. Whitney 1966–1972
Henry C. Wigley, Sr. 1955+
Frank Wilde 1958–1959+
William A. Williams, M.D. 1967–1969
Emily H. Wilson, M.D. 1951–1953
Ephraim Winer 1949–1954
William R. Woodfield 1949–1953
T. Carroll Worthington 1945–1948
Betty Wright (Mrs. John B.) 1969–1971
Harold T. Youngren 1967–196

This list of the manages and trustees of the hospital was compiled from extant minutes of the annual meetings, newspaper articles, and documents in the hospital's files. A sincere effort has been made to make it as correct as possible from the records, but there are still errors and unknowns. Additional information about these people and their terms of service would be most welcome.

The corporate reorganization in 1988 changed the title of board members from managers to trustees. Both are included here.

The chiefs and presidents of the medical staff and the presidents of the Auxiliary have been added to this list since they often attended meetings as ex officio members of the board even before these offices received voting privileges.

Names in italics indicate Chairmen of the Board.
* Members of the original Board of Managers of the Annapolis Emergency Hospital, 1902.
# Members appointed by the Summerfield Baldwin, Jr. Foundation.
+ Members appointed by the Anne Arundel County Commissioners or the Anne Arundel County Council.

Directors of the Anne Arundel Medical Center Foundation, 1984-2002

Thomas I. Baldwin
George Benson
Lou Berman D.D.S.
James D. Biles, M.D.
Stephen R. Brown, M.D.
Carl A. Brunetto
Bruce C. Burns
Anthony Calabrese, M.D.
Ree Childers
Garnett Y. Clark
Helene Colussy
Kathy Cook
Hillard Donner
Martin L. Doordan
J. Kenneth Driessen
Margaret M. Ellis
Elizabeth A. Frazier
Ruby Fuller
E.L. Gardner
Nicholas Goldsborough
Peter Gordon
Frederick Graul

Florence Greenfield
Gilbert Hardesty
Robert E. Henel, Jr.
Lisa Hillman
Richard Hochman, M.D.
Barry Jackson
Jane Jacobsen
Elizabeth M. Kingsley, M.D.
Michael LaPenta M.D.
Adm. William Lawrence
Jon Lowe, M.D.
John Lyons, M.D.
M. Lee Marston
Michael McCrudden
James McEneaney, Jr.
David S. McHold , M.D.
J. Kent McNew
Daniel W. McNew
John B. Melvin
Virginia Meredith
Charles Minter
Thomas G. Moore

James O. Olfson
Steven E. Parker
James L. Pierce
Barbara Ray
Robert T. Reeves
Geneva F. Richards
Patricia Rutemiller
Lesly Sajak
Anna Smith
Malcolm B. Smith
Maryanne Spencer
Regina Stansbury
John Suit, III
Maj. Gen. J. Francis Taylor
Carl A. TenHoopen
Carl Tenner
Leslie F. Tilghman
Lawrence W. Ulvila, Jr.
Sherburne A. Walker
Edward O. Wayson, Jr.
Fielding W. Yost
(Italics indicate Chairmen of the Board)

189

ANNE ARUNDEL MEDICAL CENTER MEDICAL BOARD, 2002

Michael S. Epstein, M.D., President
George Samaras, M.D., Vice President
Thomas Ducker, M.D., Secretary/Treasurer
Scott Burgess, M.D.
Mary Clance, M.D.
Vernon Croft, M.D.
John Danneberger, M.D.
Kenneth Gummerson, M.D.
A. Stephen Hansman, M.D.
Edward S. Holt, M.D.
Elizabeth Kingsley, M.D.
C. Daniel Laughlin, M.D.

Timothy M. Lynch, D.P.M.
Jeffrey Nold, D.O.
Michael Peters, M.D.
James W. Reinig, M.D.
Terrence L. Smith, M.D.
Clifford Solomon, M.D.
Cornelius Sullivan, D.M.D.
David R. Watt, M.D.
Michael D. Webb, M.D.
William R. Weisburger, M.D.
Debra Whitehurst-Brown, M.D.

CHIEFS AND PRESIDENTS OF THE MEDICAL STAFF, 1902-2002

W. Clement Claude, M.D. 1902-1903
George Wells, M.D. 1905-1910
James J. Murphy, M.D. 1911-1912
J. Oliver Purvis, M.D. 1914-1917
James J. Murphy, M.D. 1917-1918
J. Oliver Purvis, M.D. 1919-1920
J. Oliver Purvis, M.D. 1922-1928
James J. Murphy, M.D. 1929-1930
J. Willis Martin, M.D. 1931
Walton H. Hopkins, M.D. 1932-1935
J. Oliver Purvis, M.D. 1936
Albert Anderson, M.D. 1937
Robert S.G. Welch, M.D. 1938
J. Willis Martin, M.D. 1939
Robert S.G. Welch, M.D. 1940
Walton H. Hopkins, M.D. 1941-1944
J. Oliver Purvis, M.D. 1945
John M. Claffy, M.D. 1945-1946
Robert S.G. Welch, M.D. 1947-1949
Albert Anderson, M.D. 1951
Emily H. Wilson, M.D. 1953
Robert S.G. Welch, M.D. 1954-1956
Frank M. Shipley, M.D. 1956-1958

Manning W. Alden, M.D. 1959
John L. Hedeman, M.D. 1960-1961
J. Fred Hawkins, Jr., M.D. 1962
Barber C. Palmer, M.D. 1963-1965
Samuel Borssuck, M.D. 1965-1967
William A. Williams, M.D. 1967-1969
Richard N. Peeler, M.D. 1969-1971
Sherman S. Robinson, M.D. 1971-1973
H. Logan Holtgrewe, M.D. 1973-1975
George W. Settle, M.D. 1975-1977
Aris T. Allen, M.D. 1977-1978
Robert S. Ellis, M.D. 1978-1980
Peter F. Verkouw, M.D. 1980-1983
David S. McHold, M.D. 1983-1985
Richard I. Hochman, M.D. 1985-1987
Stephen R. Brown, M.D. 1987-1989
James D. Biles III, M.D. 1989-1991
Jon B. Lowe, M.D. 1991-1993
Anthony J. Calabrese, M.D. 1993-1995
Joseph D. Moser, M.D. 1995-1997
Michael J. LaPenta, M.D. 1997-1999
Elizabeth M. Kingsley, M.D. 1999-2001
Michael S. Epstein, M.D. 2001-present

Anne Arundel Medical Staff (January 24, 2002)

Kenneth L. Abbott, M.D.
David Brian Abell, P.A.
Charles P. Adamo, M.D.
George W. Adams, M.D.
Nadia Akhmed, M.D.
Farhad Aliabadi, M.D.
Damanhuri D. Alkaitis, M.D.
Kari M. Alperovitz-Bichell, M.D.
Jonathan A. Altschuler, M.D.
Sigmund A. Amitin, M.D.
David C. Anderson, M.D.
Clifford G. Andrew, M.D.
Nicholas H. Antoniades, M.D.
Elaine Marie Arata, M.D.
William G. Armiger, M.D.
Mariam McConnell Bahrami, M.D.
Azam Baig, M.D.
Debra L. Bailey, M.D.
Roy E. Bands, M.D.
Alpha T. Banks, M.D.
James R. Banks, M.D.
David C. Barnes, M.D.
Alison Almeida Bartfield, M.D.
Molly W. Bartlett, C.R.N.P.
Barbara L. Bean, M.D.
Sjoerd Beck, M.D.
Gregg T. Behling, D.M.D.
William E. Behrens, M.D.
Paul B. Berez, M.D.
Richard A. Bernstein, M.D.
Charles N. Bethmann, P.A.
M. Pamela Beusch, M.D.
Timothy W. Biddle, D.O.
Jessica L. Bienstock, M.D.
Wayne D. Bierbaum, M.D.
James D. Biles III, M.D.
Janice L. Bird, M.D.
James M. Blake, M.D.
Karin J. Blakemore, M.D.
Lisa Bleckner, M.D.
Larry W. Blum, M.D.
Barbara J. Blume, R.N.
Charles R. Boice, M.D.
Riaz Bokhari, M.D.
Irmina C. Boulier, M.D.
Judith L. Boyer-Patrick, M.D.

Marc F. Brassard, M.D.
Michelle E. Brayton, M.D.
Michele Elizabeth Brenner, M.D.
Marie H. Brigham, M.D.
Rodney L. Brimhall, M.D.
Konni E. Bringman, M.D.
Sandra E. Brooks, M.D.
Andrea Denise Brown, M.D.
Helen F. Brown, C.R.N.P.
Stephen D. Brown, M.D.
Steven F. Brown, M.D.
Susan Marie Brown, C.N.M.
William F. Bruther, M.D.
Jill A. Brydalski, C.R.N.P.
Warren L. Buchalter, M.D.
D. Paul Buhrer, M.D.
Scott Burgess, M.D.
Timothy Grayson Burke, M.D.
Louise C. Burns, C.R.N.P.
Anthony J. Calabrese, M.D.
Angela M. Calle, M.D.
Linda Brooks Cameron, M.D.
Patrick Joseph Canan, D.O.
Joan Cantero-Lakhanpal, M.D.
Nicholas A. Capozzoli, M.D.
Anthony M. Caputo, M.D.
Alexis J. Carras, M.D.
William A. Cassidy, M.D.
Christine G. Cattaneo, M.D.
George B. Cavanagh, M.D.
James M. Chamberlain, M.D.
Donna Gordon Chambers, M.D.
Betty Chang, M.D.
James E. Chappell, M.D.
Christian A. Chisholm, M.D.
Aditya Chopra, M.D.
Gerard Church, M.D.
Mary R. Clance, M.D.
Kevin L. Clark, M.D.
Michael R. Clemmens, M.D.
Sheri Bleacher Coleman,
   C.R.N.P.
Nilda M. Collins, D.M.D.
Hector K. Collison, M.D.
John J. Conroy, M.D.
Ajia S. Coolbaugh, R.N.

David H. Corddry, M.D.
Jane Ann Corner, C.R.N.P.
Vernon R. Croft, M.D.
Gale G. Cromwell, C.R.N.P.
Susan D. Cummings, M.D.
Patricia A. Czapp, M.D.
William A. Dabbs, M.D.
Azar Peter Dagher, M.D.
Riad Dakheel, M.D.
Stephen L. Dalton, M.D.
John E. Danneberger, M.D.
Gerri L. Davis, M.D.
Hung T. Davis, M.D.
Randy F. Davis, M.D.
Martin K. Deafenbaugh, M.D.
David H. Deaton, M.D.
Paula A. DeCandido, M.D.
Jeanne H. DeFeo, M.D.
John G. DeLeonibus, D.P.M.
Lauren J. DeLoach, M.D.
Frank Delosso, P.A.
Marlene DeMaio, M.D.
Thomas Richard Dennis, M.D.
Craig Christopher DeWolfe, M.D.
Beth G. Diamond, M.D.
Lisa A. DiMarzio, M.D.
Edward J. Distelhorst, M.D.
Andrew S. Dobin, M.D.
Michael J. Dodd, M.D.
Patricia G. Donoho, L.P.N.
Rita H. DuBoyce, M.D.
Thomas B. Ducker, M.D.
Edward J. Dudek, M.D.
Katherine K. Dunleavy, M.D.
Douglas D. Dykman, M.D.
Timothy S. Eckel, M.D.
R. Scott Eden, M.D.
Katherine S.K. Edwards, M.D.
Allen C. Egloff, M.D.
Paul T. Elder, M.D.
Ross D. Elliott, M.D.
Michael J. Elman, M.D.
James F. Elmore, M.D.
Sven Ingo Ender, M.D.
Michael S. Epstein, M.D.
Diego A. Escobosa, M.D.

Melissa Ann Esposito, M.D.
L. Kofi Essandoh, M.D.
Dina Esterowitz, M.D.
Stephen E. Faust, M.D.
Kristen Leigh Fernandez, M.D.
Victor Ferrans, M.D.
Douglas A. Finnegan, M.D.
Dwight N. Fortier, M.D.
Robert W. Frazier, M.D.
Michael R. Freedman, M.D.
Joseph N. Friend, M.D.
Elizabeth A. Fronc, M.D.
John W. Frost, Jr., M.D.
Edwin C. Fulton, M.D.
Barbara Travis Furlow, M.D.
Ruth K. Gallatin, M.D.
Robert A. Gallino, M.D.
Peiqing Gao, M.D.
Lori S. Garcia, M.D.
Richard B. Garden, D.D.S.
Meredith G. Garrett, M.D.
Abdul K. Garuba, M.D.
Jeffrey Gelfand, M.D.
Duane M. Gels, M.D.
Linda L. George, M.D.
Robert G. Gibson, M.D.
Parabh K. Gill, M.D.
Paul W. Gill, D.P.M.
Jackie L. Gilliard, M.D.
Glenn D. Gilmor, M.D.
Jacalyn G. Ginsburg, D.O.
Peter Charles Gleason, M.D.
Lisa I. Goldberg, M.D.
Andrew T. Goldstein, M.D.
Gail R. Goldstein, M.D.
Howard D. Goldstein, M.D.
Albert M. Gordon, M.D.
Andrew G. Gordon, M.D.
Victoria A. Gouze, M.D.
Christopher M. Grande, M.D.
Robert G. Graw, Jr., M.D.
Peter R. Graze, M.D.
Joan L. Greene, C.R.N.P.
Robert M. Greenfield, M.D.
Mary Beth Grotz, D.O.
Frederick H. Guckes, M.D.

Kenneth S. Gummerson, M.D.
Edith D. Gurewitsch, M.D.
Andre B. Gvozden, M.D.
Faith A. Hackett, M.D.
James B. Haddock, M.D.
Alyson L. Hall, M.D.
Dennis McCoy Hall, M.D.
Joseph A. Halpern, M.D.
Marc D. Hamburger, M.D.
Eileen Mary Hamill, M.D.
Mark P. Hamill, M.D.
Stephen C. Hamilton, M.D.
Joan S. Hammond, C.R.N.P.
Dirk Hamp, M.D.
Robert L. Handwerger, M.D.
A. Stephen Hansman, M.D.
Karen Hardart, M.D.
Debra K. Hardy-Cartwright, M.D.
Jamie L. Harms, M.D.
Thomas J. Harries, M.D.
Curtis Harris, M.D.
Brian E. Harvey, M.D.
Joanne Hasman, C.N.M.
Kenneth L. Hatch, D.P.M.
Charles Page Hatcher, M.D.
Thomas F. Hattar, M.D.
Claudia Cathleen Hays, M.D.
Gregg L. Heacock, M.D.
Nancy J. Heisel, M.D.
Robert A. Heller, M.D.
Heather J. Herman, M.D.
Robert Alan Herman, M.D.
Eric Hermansen, M.D.
Raymond G. Herzinger, M.D.
J. Laurance Hill, M.D.
Valory T. Hill, M.D.
Kenneth Steven Himmel, M.D.
Stephen J. Hittman, D.O.
Lubor Hlousek, D.M.D, M.D.
Richard I. Hochman, M.D.
Kenneth M. Hoffman, M.D.
Karl R. Holschuh, M.D.
Edward S. Holt, M.D.
L. Dean Hoover, M.D.
Sara Lanell Horton, M.D.
Barbara J. Howard, M.D.

N. Rachael Howland, M.D.
Cynthia W. Huffaker, M.D.
Jonathan S. Hunn, M.D.
Barbara A. Hutchinson, M.D.
O. Darcy Ibitoye, M.D.
Ali Ipakchi, M.D.
John D. Jackson, M.D.
Yvonne M. Jackson, M.D.
Stuart Leslie Jacobs, M.D.
David Elijah Jaller, M.D.
Donna Lynne Jasper, D.O.
Patricia P. Jett, M.D.
Lydia M. Jumamoy, M.D.
Jerrilyn M. Jutton, M.D.
Karen M. Kabat, M.D.
Brian S. Kahan, D.O.
Marie C. Kaifer-Zajdowicz, M.D.
Demetrios Kalliongis, M.D.
Stephen J. Katz, M.D.
Nancy G. Kelley, M.D.
Jacqueline Kelly, M.D.
Lisa D. Kelly, M.D.
John J. Kennedy, M.D.
Kenneth D. Keys, M.D.
Lubna Khan, M.D.
Mukul Khandelwal, M.D.
Stephen E. Killian, M.D.
Daniel William Killingsworth, M.D.
Charles E. King, M.D.
Nancy D. King, M.D.
Elizabeth M. Kingsley, M.D.
Arnold S. Kirshenbaum, M.D.
Lee A. Kleiman, M.D.
Donald M. Klein, P.A.
Wayne K. Knoll, Jr., D.P.M.
Kevin B. Knopf, M.D.
Daniel J. Konick, M.D.
Frank M. Kopack, M.D.
Susan H. Krieger, M.D.
S. David Krimins, M.D.
Priesh I. Kumar, M.D.
Stephan C. Kurylas, M.D.
James G. Lahti, M.D.
Sanjiv Lakhanpal, M.D.
Kathryn A. Lanciano, C.R.N.P.
Walter E. Landmesser, Jr., M.D.

David G. Lange, M.D.
Monique Y. Langston, D.O.
Thomas B. Lank, M.D.
Michael J. LaPenta, M.D.
Elizabeth H. Lasley, M.D.
John S. Latimer, M.D.
C. Daniel Laughlin, M.D.
Salvatore S. Lauria, M.D.
Young Joo Lee, M.D.
Chasheryl L. Leslie, M.D.
Christine Lewis, M.D.
Samuel M. Libber, M.D.
Jack R. Lichtenstein, M.D.
Yann-Yann Lin, M.D.
George E. Linhardt, Jr., M.D.
Robert G. Lisk, M.D.
Walter C. Lockhart, M.D.
Patrick D. Looney, D.D.S.
David H. Lowe, M.D.
Jon B. Lowe, M.D.
Nicole Marie Luecke, M.D.
Ronald W. Luethke, M.D.
Joan Luo, M.D.
Garrett J. Lynch, M.D.
Timothy M. Lynch, D.P.M.
Marinela Macaraeg, M.D.
Kevin M. Macready, M.D.
John W. Mahaffay, M.D.
Nicholas Harry Malakis, M.D.
Matthew J. Malta, M.D.
Bonnie R. Manning, P.A.
Ralph Michael Marcoot, D.D.S.
Yudhishtra Markan, M.D.
Gerard R. Martin, M.D.
John D. Martin, M.D.
Nicholette M. Martin, M.D.
Isidro R. Martinez, M.D.
Gina Marie Massoglia, M.D.
David E. Matteson, M.D.
Sejal G. Mattu, M.D.
William Clarence Maxted, Jr., M.D.
Elizabeth P. Maxwell-Schmidt, M.D.
Jay Aaron Mazel, M.D.
Daniel C. McCabe, M.D.
Clifton A. McClain III, M.D.
David W. McDermott, M.D.

Edward Robert McDevitt, M.D.
Jean-Paul McDonough, M.D.
James M. McKee, D.P.M.
David G. Medland, M.D.
Robert B. Meek III, M.D.
Marco A. Mejia, M.D.
Frank S. Melograna, M.D.
Sharon Marie Messics, M.D.
M. Kent Mewha, M.D.
Mary L. Michels, M.D.
Melissa J. Mikami, M.D.
Birgitta Elizabeth Miller, M.D.
Robert A. Miller, M.D.
Douglas Stewart Mitchell, M.D.
Gregory A. Mitchell, M.D.
Rhonda Michelle Mitchell, M.D.
Lyle T. Modlin, D.P.M.
Melissa M. Moen, M.D.
John Cyrus Moghtader, M.D.
Holly A. Mohr, C.R.N.P.
Michael B. Monias, M.D.
Elizabeth A. Montgomery, C.R.N.P.
David A. Mooradian, M.D.
Robert C. Moore, M.D.
Susan S. Moreland, C.R.N.P.
Christina Marie Morganti, M.D.
Edward J. Morris, M.D.
E.Joseph Morris, M.D.
Gilbert L. Mottla, M.D.
Mohamed Sameh Moubarek, M.D.
Margaret M. Mullins, M.D.
Lina Murad, M.D.
Kerry A. Murphy, R.N.
Lisa B. Murray, M.D.
Ella Catherine Murtha, P.A.
David W. Myers, M.D.
David A. Nagey, M.D.
Misti L. Neil, C.N.M.
Gerald W. Newman, M.D.
John L. Newman, M.D.
Christine Pham Nguyen, M.D.
Suzanne Willard Niemela, M.D.
Darlene M. Nixon, R.N.
Robert H. Noel, M.D.
Jeffrey T. Nold, D.O.
Lawrence A. Nurin, D.D.S.

Mirza M. Nusairee, M.D.
Suzanne A. E. Ochs, P.A.
Proinnsias O'Croinin, M.D.
George Joseph Odell, M.D.
Terrence Michael O'Donovan, M.D.
Patricia A. O'Hora, M.D.
Kevin J. O'Keefe, M.D.
Marcia V. Ormsby, M.D.
J. Kevin O'Rourke, M.D.
Myrna Malan Ortega, M.D.
Peter N. Ove, M.D.
David A. Paad, C.N.M.
Elba M. Pacheco, M.D.
Daina B. Pack, M.D.
Stephanie Ann Pakula
J. Michael Pardo, M.D.
Juan M. Pardo, M.D.
Steven H. Parker, M.D.
Charles Livingston Parmele, M.D.
Judith E. Parsley, C.N.M.
Mark O'Brien Peeler, M.D.
Susan Kathleen Todd Peeler, M.D.
Marcus L. Penn, M.D.
Angela R. Peterman, M.D.
Michael N. Peters, M.D.
Robert T. Peterson, M.D.
Charles Wesley Phelps, M.D.
Errol A. Phillip, M.D.
Mark D. Phillips, M.D.
Karen M. Pipkin, C.R.N.P.
Catherine R. Platnick, P.A.
Agnieszka Zofia Pluta, M.D.
Richard M. Podolin, Ph.D.
Kathleen Valentovish Potter, P.A.
David M. Powell, M.D.
Carol A. Pressey, M.D.
Webra Price-Douglas, C.R.N.P.
Lawrence S. Prichep, M.D.
Steven G. Proshan, M.D.
Robert William Raden, M.D.
Paula A. Radon, M.D.
Mark S. Radowich, M.D.
Phyllis M. Rattey, C.N.M.
Joan K. Rehner, C.R.N.P.
Deborah A. Reid, M.D.
James William Reinig, M.D.

ANNE ARUNDEL MEDICAL STAFF (CONTINUED)

C. Michael Remoll, M.D.
Lisa Joy Renfro, M.D.
Mark L. Repka, M.D.
Steven Craig Resnick, M.D.
Paul S. Rhodes, M.D.
James William Rice, M.D.
Michael S. Riebman, M.D.
Marie Suzanne Rindfleisch, D.O.
James L. Rivers, Jr., M.D.
Jane P. Roach, C.R.N.P.
Donald C. Roane, M.D.
Elizabeth L. Robbins, M.D.
Sanford H. Robbins III, M.D.
Clare Marie T. Rodgers, C.R.N.P.
Paul D. Rogers, M.D.
William Herman Rogers, M.D.
Frank Hancock Roland, Jr., M.D.
Christopher A. Roseberry, M.D.
Martin J. Rosenberg, M.D.
James W. Ross, M.D.
Sharon A. Rowe, L.P.N.
Arnon Erez Rubin, M.D.
Cheryl A. Ruddick, C.R.N.P.
Jonathan Brett Rudick, M.D.
Charles M. Ruland, M.D.
Louis Joseph Ruland III, M.D.
James W. Ruppel, M.D.
Parviz Sahandy, M.D.
Sanjiv K. Saini, M.D.
Eric A. Salata, M.D.
George C. Samaras, M.D.
Suzanne L. Sankey, M.D.
Geoffrey H. Saunders, M.D.
T. Richard Saunders, Ph.D.
Vincent F. Sayan, M.D.
Janine Sayles, C.N.M.
Ricardo L. Scartascini, M.D.
Vannesa Viviana Scartascini, P.A.
Cynthia Niemeyer Schaeffer, M.D.
Lawrence S. Schieken, M.D.
Peter Schilder, M.D.
Elizabeth Louise Schilling, C.R.N.P.
Patrick P. Schimpf, M.D.
Jeffrey Clark Schmidlein, M.D.
Donald R. Schneider, M.D.
Christopher F. Schultz, M.D.

Arthur H. Schwartz, M.D.
Mitchell B. Schwartz, M.D.
Netanel G. Schwob, M.D.
Maria C. Scott, M.D.
Matthew J. Scott, M.D.
Ramona G. Seidel, M.D.
Stuart E. Selonick, M.D.
Elizabeth Frances Shade, M.D.
Sandra C. Shanahan, C.R.N.P.
Perry Shipley Shelton, M.D.
Henry L. Sherwood, M.D.
Rochelle DiZio Shin, M.D.
Mahmaud Shirazi, M.D.
Daljeet Singh Sidhu, M.D.
Patricia Ann Simmons, C.R.N.P.
Michael R. Singleton, M.D.
Ryszard Skulski, M.D.
Michele R. Smadja-Gordon, M.D.
Randy Smargiassi, D.P.M.
Debra Ann Smith, C.R.N.P.
Garth R. Smith, M.D.
Stephen R. Smith, P.A.
Terence L. Smith, M.D.
Jeremy S. Snow, M.D.
Henry J. Sobel, M.D.
Clifford Todd Solomon, M.D.
Joydeep Som, M.D.
Helen Song, C.R.N.P.
Cynthia M. Soriano, M.D.
Alessandro Constantino Speciale, M.D.
Christopher Joseph Spittler, M.D.
Gary J. Sprouse, M.D.
Ronald C. Sroka, M.D.
Michol Stanzione, D.O.
Kimberly A. Stauffer, C.R.N.P.
Marshall K. Steele III, M.D.
Harvey J. Steinfeld, M.D.
Peter F. Stengel, M.D.
Daniel E. Stenger, P.A.
Eric D. Strauch, M.D.
Carl W. Strawberry, M.D.
Theresa L. Strong, C.R.N.P.
Raymond Arthur Sturner, M.D.
Brian J. Sullivan, M.D.
Cornelius J. Sullivan, D.M.D.
Kelley W. Sullivan, M.D.

Adam N. Summers, M.D.
Gyan Chand Surana, M.D.
Frederick Thomas Sutter, M.D.
Peter A. Swaby, D.O.
Lorraine Tafra, M.D.
Barry S. Tatar, M.D.
Nader Tavakoli-Jalili, M.D.
William Tham, M.D.
Michelle Denise Thomas, M.D.
Kerry J. Thompson, M.D.
Roseanne K. Thompson, C.R.N.P.
Denise Kristin Thurling, M.D.
Krystal V. Tibbs, C.R.N.P.
Clark Jiro Tingleaf, M.D.
Brad A. Toll, D.P.M.
David J. Tolner, M.D.
Angel E. Torano, M.D.
Donna M. Trageser, C.R.N.P.
C. Jay Tull III, D.D.S.
Oguz Y. Turgut, M.D.
Margaret Catherine Turner, M.D.
Ira Mark Tyler, M.D.
Barbara Tymkiw, M.D.
Chukwuemeka C. Ufomadu, M.D.
Emily A. Ulmer, M.D.
Barbara P. Urban, M.D.
Emil Frank Valle, M.D.
Linda Kanz Vanderslice, M.D.
Jack J. VanGeffen, M.D.
Julia A. VanHassent, P.A.
Denise Varquez-Hoffman, D.P.M.
Julia Lombard Venuti, C.R.N.P.
Rose M. VerElst, M.D.
Robert M. Verklin, Jr., M.D.
Rebecca Vickers, M.D.
William E. Vickers, M.D.
Roger W. Voigt, M.D.
Cuong D. Vu, M.D.
A. Terry Walman, M.D.
Thomas M. Walsh, M.D.
Clifford S. Walzer, D.M.D.
Earl C. Wang, M.D.
James W. Wang, M.D.
Jean Warner, M.D.
Stanley P. Watkins, Jr., M.D.
Randall W. Watson, P.A.

David R. Watt, M.D.
Michael David Webb, M.D.
Stanley R. Weimer, M.D.
Ira Martin Weinstein, M.D.
David Charles Weintritt, M.D.
William R. Weisburger, M.D.
Richard G. Welch, M.D.
Barbara Gail Wells, M.D.
Barry H. Wells, M.D.
Jeanine L. Werner, M.D.
Stephan Lionel Werner, M.D.
Milton W. Werthmann, M.D.
Shannon L. West, M.D.
Sarah M. White, M.D.

Debora V. Whitehurst-Brown, M.D.
John H. Wilckens, M.D.
Joh F. Wiley, M.D.
Jon E. Williams, Ph.D.
Alan F. Wolf, M.D.
Anthony B. Wolff, Ph.D.
Loyd A. Wolfley, M.D.
Timothy Gerard Woods, M.D.
Joan E. Woodward, M.D.
Misty Lee Wray, M.D.
Jodi Lynne Wright, R.N.
Eric A. Wulfsberg, M.D.
Ellen Y. Yang, M.D.
James J. York, M.D.

Mary Elizabeth Young, M.D.
Aimee Y. Yu, M.D.
George W. Yu, M.D.
Miriam M. Yudkoff, M.D.
Melinda Zagarino, R.N.
Edward M. Zagula, M.D.
S. Sohail Zaidi, M.D.
Bulent Zaim, M.D.
Burger Zapf, M.D.
Edward Zebovitz, D.D.S.
Nano Zeringue, M.D.
Susan Zimmerman, M.D.
Lawrence P. Zyskowski, M.D.

Anne Arundel Medical Center
Auxiliary Board of Directors
Executive Committee, 2002

Katherine Cook, President
Kathryn Clabby, 1st Vice President
Rebecca Quattlebaum, 2nd Vice President
Judy Hall, 3rd Vice President
Joan P. Kelly, Recording Secretary

Sara Ostrusky, Treasurer
Ida Marshall, Financial Secretary
Nan Terhorst, Corresponding Secretary
Barbara Ray, Past President

Presidents of the Hospital
Auxiliary, 1942-2002

Selda V. Miller 1944-1946
Charlotte Borssuck 1947-1948
Beatrice Hiltabidle 1949-1950
Mrs. C. Addison Hodges 1950-1951
Jeanette Joachim 1951-1952
Ethel Corbin 1952-1954
Jean M. Deghee 1954-1956
Ruth Boro 1956-1958
Bernadine Sheehan 1958-1960
Charlotte Brown 1960-1961
Isabel Murray 1961-1963
Nancy Gideon 1963-1965
Rebecca M. Clatanoff 1965-1967
Irma Myers 1967-1969
Betty Wright 1969-1971
Margaret Hood 1971-1972

Louise Morris 1973-1974
Ruth Schnell 1974-1976
Jean Meehla 1976-1978
Geraldine Settle 1978-1980
Janet Bauer 1980-1981
Anna Smith 1981-1983
Geneva F. Richards 1983-1985
Ruby Fuller 1985-1987
Margaret M. Ellis 1987-1989
Ree Childers 1989-1991
Jane Jacobsen 1991-1993
Nancy Headley 1993-1994
Regina Stansbury 1994-1996
Patricia Rutemiller 1996-1998
Barbara Ray 1998-2000
Katherine Cook, 2000-2002

Administrators & Presidents of Anne Arundel Medical Center, 1945-2002

Loran S. Messick 1944–1946
Sherrill S. Adams 1947–1956
Charles S. Smisson 1956–1958*
Lyman C. Whittaker 1958–1979

Carl A. Brunetto 1979–1988
Martin L. Doordan 1988–present

*Acting administrator

Superintendents of Annapolis Emergency Hospital, 1902-1944

(in chronological order)
Nellie M. Pusey
Ruth A. E. Adamson
Etta S. H. Rayle
Millicent Geare
Rosamond Minnis
Alice T. Bell
Margaret Wohlgemuth
Mary K. Geraci
E. E. Welty
Miss Hollinger

Eleanor Saffer
Margaret Wohlgemuth
E. Blanche Hoffmeister
Margaret M. Judge
Ruth Rhodes
Elizabeth Gallery
Ruth Clements
Katherine V. Shea
Mabel Merrick
Marie Stein
Ada Mae Leitch

THE FIRST 90 YEARS
(CHAPTERS 1-7)

Jane W. McWilliams

A great many people helped with the research and production of *The First 90 Years* in 1992, and they were acknowledged fully in that publication. The administration, physicians, nurses and staff of the hospital at the time were unfailingly cooperative, among them Carl Brunetto, Martin L. Doordan, Lisa Hillman and Fran D. Counihan and the hospital's public relations staff.

Oral histories taken in 1991 under the auspices of the Center for the Study of Local Issues at the Anne Arundel Community College were important to the first book, as were interviews I conducted in 1992. Those who contributed their memories and knowledge of the hospital included Dr. Faye Allen, Dr. Philip Briscoe, Helen M. Cirillo, Rebecca M. Clatanoff, Ann Cole, Shirley H. Fuller, R.N., Cassie Gaskins, Beatrice Hiltabidle, Marguerite Labrot-Spence, William J. McWilliams, Dr. Richard N. Peeler, Dr. Frank M. Shipley, Dr. Stanley P. Watkins, Jr., Lyman C. Whittaker, Dr. Emily Wilson and Lucille Worthington.

The staff of the Nimitz Library at the U.S. Naval Academy; James Cheevers of the Naval Academy Museum; William E. Taylor of the Navy's Chaplain Resource Board; Arian Ravanbakhsh of the Alan Mason Chesney Medical Archives at Johns Hopkins Hospital; Nancy Bramucci, Susan Cummings, Teresa Fountain, Jim Hefelfinger, Phebe Jacobsen, Gregory Stiverson and Mame Warren at the Maryland State Archives; Isabel Cunningham of Calvary Methodist Church; Robert Worden of St. Mary's Church; Nancy Osius of St. John's College; Gillian Barr of Historic Annapolis Foundation; Mrs. Bruce A. Beckner of the DAR; Charles W. White of the Elks Club; Adam Sczetaniuak of the Medical and Chirurgical Society of Maryland; Adrienne Noe and Ralph Hawk of the Walter Reed Army Hospital, and the public relations staffs of six other community hospitals in Maryland all offered valuable assistance or information.

Additional information came from Dr. Alex Boro, Peg Burroughs, Ree Childers, Joyce Disharoon, Michael Kaiser, Tony Lindauer, William J. McWilliams, Jr., Mary Meekins, Virginia Meredith, Anna Monias, Virginia Schaun, Florence Seaman, R.N., Frank C. Serio and Katherine H. Trettin.

Photographs and memorabilia for the book were found in the hospital's files, in public institutions such as the Maryland State Archives and in private collections. Ruth Boro, Dr. Gerard Church, Helen Simmons Cirillo, Rebecca Clatanoff, Ann Cole, Mary Gray Crandall, Margaret Ellis, Shirley H. Fuller, R.N., Sally Welch Geary, Jane H. Jacobsen, Katherine Tyler Jones, Marguerite Labrot-Spence, Berry Lowman, John W. Martin III, Doris R. Moses, Emily H. Peake, Dr. Richard N. Peeler, Geneva Richards, Lin Rizzo, Mary A. Russell, Susie B. Stewart, Lyman C. Whittaker, Dr. Emily Wilson, and Jean and Jake Wohlgemuth gave permission for the use of their treasured photographs or offered information for captions.

Production of the first book was made possible by the assistance of Ann Hofstra Grogg, editor; Peg Udall, designer; Joan Albert, Rhea Claggett, Lynne MacAdam and Christine Scanlon. Anne Arundel Orthopedic Surgeons, Inc. provided an office for the project, and Madeleine Hughes was both research assistant and support team.

My thanks to all these people, some now deceased, for their contributions 10 years ago. They made this book happen, too.

Acknowledgments

A Century of Caring
(Chapters 8-9 and Perspectives)

Catherine H. Avery

Like all achievements at Anne Arundel Medical Center, the writing of the final two chapters and the production of this new book was a team effort. Members of the hospital family enthusiastically participated, including administrators, physicians, nurses and others. Each member of the public relations staff played an important role, especially Mary Lou Baker, Lisa Hillman, Martha Harlan and Devon Madden. A very special thanks goes to book designer Bob Madden for making this history come alive.

Much of the material was derived from the board's meeting minutes, past issues of *Vital Signs*, back issues of *The Capital*, public relations files and firsthand observation of recent events. But what gave the facts depth was the participation of many individuals who played vital roles in the growth of the hospital. These people included Chip Doordan, Lisa Hillman, Chuck Brunetto, Dr. Joseph Moser, Jock Hopkins, Carolyn Core, Dennis Curl and Beth Evins, all of whom gave generously of their time and knowledge about the last decade and the preceding years. Administration members Sharon Riley and George Blair also participated and Michelle Harder ably compiled statistics.

Charlie Steele cheerfully led me on tours of the new hospital at several key junctures, while Joan Kelly helped familiarize me with the old hospital. Behind the scenes, Lin Rizzo and Sally Morris made my job easier throughout the months of preparation, and Norma Babington, Philip Rink, Jr., Justus Burkhardt and Michelle Bennett hunted for photographs. Many physicians provided information about the hospital's programs, including Dr. Vernon Croft, Dr. Elizabeth Kingsley, Dr. Michael LaPenta, Dr. Clifford Solomon, Dr. Marshall K. Steele III and Dr. Stanley P. Watkins, Jr. Other employees who participated included Kris Powell and Karen Peddicord, along with a host of others.

Board members James McEneaney, Jr. and Becki Kurdle offered their input, as did Foundation leaders Hillard Donner and George Benson and Auxilian Barbara Ray. Former County Executive John Gary shared his perceptions, as did publisher Philip Merrill.

Selected community members agreed to interviews and photographs that provided invaluable "Perspectives" throughout the book. These included Peg Burroughs, Dr. Emily Wilson, Bee Hiltabidle, Dr. Frank Shipley, Dr. Faye Allen, Chuck Brunetto, Dr. Richard Peeler, Nancy Achenback, Jock Hopkins and Chip Doordan.

Finally, the Centennial Book Committee offered guidance throughout the book's development. Members included Nancy Achenback, Mary Lou Baker, Chuck Brunetto, Chip Doordan, Martha Harlan, Lisa Hillman, Jock Hopkins, Irma Myers, Dr. Richard Peeler, Bob Rich and Charlie Steele.

Many thanks to all.

Photography and Illustration Credits

Sources

Anne Arundel Medical Center, 20, 35, 37, 43, 48, 51, 56, 59, 60 below, 70, 77, 79 below, 80 below, 87, 88 below, 95, 96, 103, 104, 109, 111, 115, 119, 120, 122, 124, 130, 131, 133, 139, 140, 141, 144, 145, 146, 149, 150, 151, 152, 153, 154, 157, 158 above, 163, 164, 169, 179
Cirillo, Helen Simmons, 36
Cole, Ann, 80
Crandall, Mary Gray, 50, 60 above
Crosby Communications, 138
Cunningham, Isabel S., 6
Evening Capital, 66, 73, 76, 85, 89, 90, 91, 93, 99, 106, 107, 112, 113, 114, 123, 126, 127, 129, 137, 154
Geary, Sally Welch, 21
Holland-Peake, Emily, 25
James R. Edmunds Jr. Architects, 72
Jones, Katherine Tyler, 48
Madison Homes, 159
Martin, John, 58
Maryland State Archives [MSA SC 1878], 40, 42
Maryland State Archives, Rowland Meade Collection [MSA SC 1672], 54
Maryland State Archives, Moses Collection [MSA SC 1465], 26
Maryland State Archives, Pickering Negatives Collection [MSA SC 1936], 61
Maryland State Archives, Marion Warren Collection [MSA SC 1890], 19, 29, 56, 74, 79 above, 80 above
Washington Post, 86
West Annapolis Volunteer Fire Department, 45
Whelan, Stu, 98
Whittaker, Lyman C., 88 above
Wilson, Dr. Emily, 52

Photographers and Illustrators

Baer, John, 72
Barton-Gillet Co., 87
Del Vecchio, Charles, 86
Edhal, Edward J., 99, 106
Gilbert, Bob, 123, 129
Gillis, John, 154
Gruver, Joe, 112
Hambrock, Charles Wallace, 45
Lundskow, George "Nick", 168
Max MacKenzie, 10 below left, right,center, 143
Madden, Robert, 170, 172, 173, 175, 176, 177
Meade, Rowland, 56, 59, 54
Miller, Roger, 159 above
Molesky, Mark, 7, 9, 10, 11, 12, 13, 14, 15, 145, 150, 151, 152, 153, 158 below, 160, 163, 164, 169 below, 179
Odell, Mark M., 137
Pease, Greg, 122
Pickering, Edgar H. , 61
Rubino, Joe, 124 below
Twin Lens Photo, 8
Volcjak, Bill, 133, 146, 157
Westegren, Dan, 17, 22, 27, 33, 38, 41, 47, 57, 58, 63, 65, 73, 76, 83, 91, 101, 105, 110, 117, 135, 167
Whelan, Stu, 89, 93, 98,
Warren, Marion E., 74, 79 above, 80 above

Thanks to the following medical staff members who lent items from their collections of antique medical instruments for use as design elements in this book: Dr. Gerard Church, Dr. Michael S. Epstein, Dr. Elizabeth Maxwell-Schmidt, Rebecca Mikesell Byrd, R.N. and Dr. Richard N. Peeler. Other design elements were provided by Paul Vitale, Pharm.D. and borrowed from the archives of Anne Arundel Medical Center.

Catherine H. Avery

Author, Chapters 8-9 and the Perspectives

Catherine Avery moved to Annapolis in 1994 after 20 years in Washington, D.C. and Northern Virginia. She has specialized in writing about health care and medical topics for the past 15 years, following stints as a technology writer and journalist. Ms. Avery has written numerous materials for hospitals throughout the Baltimore-Washington area, the Maryland Hospital Association and a variety of publications. A native New Englander, she is a graduate of Syracuse University. She and her husband live near Thomas Point and have one son in Los Angeles.

Jane W. McWilliams

Author, Chapters 1-7

A native Annapolitan, Jane Wilson McWilliams has been researching local history for more than 35 years. She is a graduate of Washington College and for 17 years was a member of the research staff of the Maryland State Archives. In addition to her research on land and people for private clients, Ms. McWilliams has written or edited numerous publications on Maryland and Annapolis history. Her books include *Bay Ridge on the Chesapeake* (1986), which she co-authored with Carol Patterson, and *The First 90 Years* (1992). Ms. McWilliams is currently working on a history of Annapolis. She has two children, both born in the downtown hospital, and one grandchild.

Colophon

Color separations and duotones by
Chroma Graphics, Inc., Largo, Maryland

Typography in Adobe Garamond and Optima

Printed by Chroma Graphics, Inc., Largo,
Maryland on Gleneagle 100 lb. Gloss text

Smyth-Sewn bindings
American Trade Bindery, Baltimore, Maryland

Design
Robert W. Madden

Published by Anne Arundel Medical Center
February 2002

Index